Pathways of Care

Pathways of Care

EDITED BY

SUE JOHNSON
BSc (Hons) RGN, PGCEA, RNT

Blackwell
Science

© 1997 by
Blackwell Science Ltd
Editorial Offices:
Osney Mead, Oxford OX2 0EL
25 John Street, London WC1N 2BL
23 Ainslie Place, Edinburgh EH3 6AJ
350 Main Street, Malden
  MA 02148 5018, USA
54 University Street, Carlton
  Victoria 3053, Australia
10, rue Casimir Delavigne
  75006 Paris, France

Other Editorial Offices:

Blackwell Wissenschafts-Verlag GmbH
Kurfürstendamm 57
10707 Berlin, Germany

Blackwell Science KK
MG Kodenmacho Building
7–10 Kodenmacho Nihombashi
Chuo-ku, Tokyo 104, Japan

First published 1997
Reprinted 1999, 2000

Set in 11/13 pt Ehrhardt
by DP Photosetting, Aylesbury, Bucks
Printed and bound in Great Britain by
MPG Books Ltd, Bodmin, Cornwall

The Blackwell Science logo is a trade mark
of Blackwell Science Ltd, registered at the
United Kingdom Trade Marks Registry

DISTRIBUTORS

Marston Book Services Ltd
PO Box 269
Abingdon
Oxon OX14 4YN
(Orders: Tel: 01235 465500
         Fax: 01235 465555)

USA
Blackwell Science, Inc.
Commerce Place
350 Main Street
Malden, MA 02148 5018
(Orders: Tel: 800 759 6102
              781 388 8250
         Fax: 781 388 8255)

Canada
Login Brothers Book Company
324 Saulteaux Crescent
Winnipeg, Manitoba R3J 3T2
(Orders: Tel: 204 837 2987
         Fax: 204 837 3116)

Australia
Blackwell Science Pty Ltd
54 University Street
Carlton, Victoria 3053
(Orders: Tel: 03 9347 0300
         Fax: 03 9347 5001)

A catalogue record for this title
is available from the British Library
ISBN 0–632–04076–9

Library of Congress
Cataloging-in-Publication Data

Pathways of care/edited by Sue Johnson.
    p. cm.
    Includes bibliographical references and index.
    ISBN 0-632-04076-9
    1. Nursing—Great Britain—Quality control.
    2. Critical path analysis.   I. Johnson, Sue, RGN.
    [DNLM: 1. Critical Pathways. 2. Nursing Care.
    WY 100 P294 1996]
    RT85.5.P365   1996
    610.73'0941—dc20
    DNLM/DLC
    for Library of Congress   96-28014
                                              CIP

For further information on
Blackwell Science, visit our website:
www.blackwell-science.coms

Contents

Foreword

Peter Griffiths
Deputy Chief Executive, King's Fund

I was pleased to be invited to write the Foreword to this comprehensive text that provides an explanation of a new and innovative tool, Pathways of Care. Such new methods that challenge the way we manage the delivery of healthcare, both clinically and non-clinically, must be widely considered and honestly reviewed. The use of the Pathway tool is growing at a tremendous rate across the United Kingdom, and is increasingly being developed within health care settings around the world. The Pathways illustrated in this book will provide useful models for those charged with the co-ordination of care.

This book covers what the tool Pathways of care is all about, how it is used in both the acute and non-acute settings, and what it offers us when facing the many issues of today's health care (automation of records, legal aspects of records and care, risk management, contracting processes, clinical effectiveness, evidence supported practice integrated into clinical practice, cost effectiveness of treatments, outcome measurement, standard monitoring). The text is flowing and clear, making *Pathways of Care* an easy to read, accessible book.

It is essential reading for all involved in quality, effective patient care management, documentation reviews, from both the clinical and management professions. It is also an important text for those investigating any form of case management, new possibilities with the system of costing and contracting for care, and continuous quality improvement.

It is particularly pleasing that the book draws from the experience of many contributors from a variety of acute and non-acute sites in this country and overseas. I would draw attention to the chapters covering the major issues of a health service entering the twenty-first century: automation of Pathways, using Pathways in the contracting process, legal issues, litigation relating to the Pathway tool and risk management.

I welcome *Pathways of Care* as a much awaited explanation of a new tool, that will promote interest, debate and honest consideration of the Pathway system.

Preface

Sue Johnson

Pathways of Care have been used in the United Kingdom for over five years, yet to date there is little written on the topic by British Pathway users. The wealth of information on Pathways comes from the USA, where Caremaps® or Critical Paths have been used for some time. There is a need for new British texts on Pathways as their use in the UK differs in some ways from that in the States, where the health-insurance-based health care system is driven by the need for cost-effective care that delivers expected outcomes in an efficient manner. Pathways in that kind of system have a role to play in co-ordinating and controlling care to contain costs. In contrast Pathways of Care in the UK are predominantly used as a quality improvement tool with the aim of improving multidisciplinary teamworking, integrating clinical guidelines into practice, and monitoring standards and outcomes in relation to the care practices employed. In this way, Pathways of Care are a major tool for enabling clinical effectiveness.

The use of Pathways in the UK needs to be explained and this text sets out to do just that. Part 1 explains the Pathway tool; Parts 2 and 3 give real examples of Pathways being used in acute, community and mental health settings from many sites around the country; Part 4 considers the wider issues facing the National Health Service today and how Pathways have a central role to play in the future of care delivery, including risk management, legal aspects of documentation, contracting, and automation of records.

Many claims are made of Pathways: that they can reduce costs, reduce lengths of stay and improve the quality of patient care. Many sites can show local evidence of such claims, but set in isolation, these examples are purely anecdotal. However, provision of health care today is required to be evidence-based and to demonstrate clinical effectiveness. There is a national need for sound research on the use of Pathways of Care and the resulting changes that they appear to facilitate; how can we ethically endorse a tool to integrate evidence into practice, if that tool is itself not based on evidence that it is effective?

The management of health care delivery is changing, as new treatments and systems of funding arise. In this state of flux, there is a need for new ways of reviewing and co-ordinating the processes and outcomes of patient care; Pathways of Care offer an innovative and exciting prospect for health care management for the 1990s and beyond, and demand to be investigated by all providers, purchasers and users of health care services.

List of Contributors

John S. Belstead, *MB, FRCSEd, FRCSEd Orth, FFAEM*
Consultant, Accident and Emergency, Ashford Hospital NHS Trust, Ashford, Middlesex

Janet Brereton, *RGN, BSc (Hons) Nursing*
Formerly Integrated Care Pathways Co-ordinator, Charing Cross Hospital, London

Brian W. Ellis, *MB, FRCS*
Consultant Urologist, Ashford Hospital NHS Trust, Ashford, Middlesex

Garry A. Favor,
Project Leader, Baptist Health System, Birmingham, Alabama and Consulting Associate for the Center of Case Management, South Natick, Massachusetts, USA

Alison Harper, *RGN, RSCN, NATC, Dip Asthma Care*
Paediatric Ward Sister, Merlin Ward, Ashford Hospital NHS Trust, Ashford, Middlesex

Elizabeth Ann Higginson, *RGN, Dip/Cert Gerontology*
Formerly Acting Nurse Adviser and Project Manager, Hospital at Home, Hounslow and Spelthorne Community and Mental Health NHS Trust, Hounslow, Middlesex

Susan Huckle, *BA, RGN*
Formerly Senior Nurse Cardiac Directorate, St Mary's NHS Trust, London

Sue Johnson, *BSc (Hons), RGN, PGCEA, RNT*
Independent Consultant. Formerly Integrated Care Pathways Facilitator, Ashford Hospital NHS Trust, Ashford, Middlesex

Denise Kitchiner, *MD, MRCP*
Consultant in Paediatric Cardiology, Royal Liverpool Children's NHS Trust, Liverpool

Rebecca E. Ricks, *MSN, RN*
Clinical Consultant/Advisor, Baptist Health System, Birmingham,

Alabama, and Consulting Associate for the Center of Case Management, South Natick, Massachusetts, USA

Louise M. Stead, *RGN, Dip (Health Management)*
Senior Nurse, Professional Development Team, St Mary's NHS Trust, London

Thoreya Swage, *MBBS (Lond), MA (Oxon)*
Independent Health Care Consultant. Formerly Director of Primary Care Development, West Surrey Health Authority, Camberley, Surrey

Karen Thornborrow, *RGN*
Sister, Accident and Emergency Department, Ashford Hospital NHS Trust, Ashford, Middlesex

Jenny Thornton, *MCSP, SRP, Dip (Physiotherapy)*
Independent Management Consultant. Formerly Care Group Manager, Child and Adolescent Psychiatry, Hounslow and Spelthorne Community Mental Health NHS Trust, Hounslow, Middlesex

John Tingle, *BA (Law Hons), CertEd, MEd, Barrister*
Reader in Health Law and Director of the Centre for Health Law, Nottingham Law School, The Nottingham Trent University, and Visiting Professor of Law, Loyola University, Chicago, USA

Kenneth A. Walker, *MB, FRCS*
Consultant Orthopaedic and Trauma Surgeon, Ashford Hospital NHS Trust, Ashford, Middlesex

Jo Wilson, *MSc, PG Dip, BSc (Hons), MIPD, AIRM, MHSM, RGN, RM, RSCN*
Director, Healthcare Risk Resources International, Newcastle upon Tyne, and Visiting Lecturer/Practitioner, Centre for Health Law, The Nottingham Trent University

Part 1

The Pathway Tool

Chapter 1

Introduction to Pathways of Care

Sue Johnson

Introduction

The British National Health Service (NHS) is one of the largest employers in Europe. Any large business or organisation, whether providing a service or delivering a product, must have some kind of formal structure to function effectively. The larger the organisation, the more important the need for proper structured processes, procedures and policies. Within the NHS, we are delivering a very important and complex service to many thousands of patients, customers or users. Certainly the users of the NHS want all within that service to work towards providing the best possible outcomes of care and treatment. In order to do that the NHS must have a solid structure, with sound policies that extend throughout the whole of the service.

Priorities in the provision of health care are decided by the local purchasing authorities, based on an assessment of local health need. Yet to implement such policies, the structure of the NHS must include sound procedures for certain activities and treatments, and must also ensure that there is a means of 'controlling' the processes of care delivery. Each hospital or community unit needs a method by which it can identify and then evaluate its processes of care delivery so that such processes may be updated and improved upon in order that the user's outcomes may in turn be improved. Pathways of Care have much to offer the NHS as a tool for identifying, evaluating and then modifying processes of care delivery.

The use of Pathways of Care is rapidly gaining popularity throughout the United Kingdom. In 1996 over 80 NHS trusts were either piloting the use of Pathways or had fully implemented Pathways programmes. Pathways of Care are being used in all areas of health care: acute, community, mental health, maternity, adult and paediatric. Part 2 of this book gives the reader examples of Pathways being used in different settings, from acute surgery to community mental health, to demonstrate that using a Pathway scheme is not confined to the acute hospital surgical setting as many seem to believe.

Pathways may be applied to any speciality or setting within our health service.

However, despite the recent increases in the use of Pathways, it must be highlighted that there is little, if any, scientific research to support or refute their use. Most sites pilot their use based on anecdotal success stories from other Pathway user sites. As a National Health Service we are overdue in commissioning valid research to comprehensively evaluate the use of Pathways.

In this text we use 'Pathways of Care' as a generic term to cover all the different applications of Pathways, which come under many labels from protocols and guidelines to maps (Fig. 1.1). The name each health care provider organisation chooses to use is determined locally to facilitate acceptance of the programme by local clinical staff. The reader will notice throughout this text that local acceptance or ownership of a Pathway programme is crucial to its success. Any programme that involves changes in the practices and processes of care delivery must be accepted by the staff involved in, and affected by, that programme or progress may be severely hindered. Hence it is appropriate that names are chosen that are locally acceptable and not misinterpreted by the staff using the programme.

Integrated Care Pathways (ICPs)
Anticipated Recovery Pathways (ARPs)
Multidisciplinary Pathways of Care (MPCs)
Care Protocols
Critical Pathways
Care Maps®

Fig. 1.1   Different names used for Pathways of Care.

For example, many acute NHS trusts originally used the term Anticipated Recovery Pathways (ARPs), which was appropriate when applying Pathway methods to the recovery of surgical cases. The word 'anticipated' was useful as it indicated that the Pathways were planned in advance or in anticipation of the care being delivered. However, once many of these acute Pathway programmes extended into medicine and elderly care, 'recovery' was no longer viewed as a suitable description of the type of care delivered by the multidisciplinary teams involved. The emphasis of such programmes was, and is, on the integration of all the different disciplines to work together as a team, so the term 'Integrated Care Pathway' (ICP) has been substituted in many sites.

'Pathways of Care' is used in this book to cover all the other names used by different sites around the UK.

Pathways as a tool

Pathways of Care are a tool. When a workman sets out to build a wall, he uses a tool to mix the cement, and then to apply the cement between the bricks. The workman uses the tool in the way he wants. He is in control of the tool, and he also controls the work performed through the use of this tool. The tool cannot dictate to the workman what he should do and how he should do it. In the same way, Pathways of Care are a tool, and the health care delivery teams are the workmen. The health care delivery teams are in control of the Pathway tool, and the Pathways may be adapted by those teams so that they are an appropriate tool for the setting within which they are being used.

Pathways of Care are a concept, not a fixed method cast in stone. Hence the manifestation of a Pathway as a written document is individual for each site using them. This is clearly demonstrated in Parts 2 and 3 of the book where the reader will see examples of Pathways from many different settings.

As a tool, Pathways will facilitate continuous improvement in the quality of patient care. They provide a mechanism for reviewing the processes, practices and outcomes of care delivery, leading on to the improvement and upgrading of such processes and practices, resulting in better patient outcomes and a higher quality of patient care. Thus Pathways of Care are a Continuous Quality Improvement (CQI) activity, in its simplest form, applied directly to patient care.

Figure 1.2 shows a classic quality cycle. In order to improve quality, within whichever context you are working, one must start by reviewing current practices, procedures and processes of care delivery that are employed. This would involve reviewing procedure books and practice

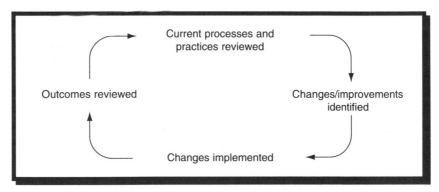

Fig. 1.2   A classic quality cycle.

guidelines to see if they are up to date, relevant, research-based and appropriately used in clinical practice. From such reviews changes and improvements are identified, which may involve redrafts of procedures and guidelines, or changes in the processes of care delivery; for example, starting up a pre-admission clinic for elective surgery patients, or commencing oral feeding a day earlier after oral surgery. Once such improvements are identified, they then need to be implemented and allowed to run for a period of time, after which the outcomes are reviewed to see if the changes have had a positive impact on the outcomes of care.

This type of quality cycle system can be applied to the use of Pathways (Fig. 1.3). A Pathway is written for a specific case-type by a multi-disciplinary team. The team reviews the current processes, procedures, guidelines and practices of care delivery and sets them out as a Pathway. The Pathway is implemented and then every 30–50 cases the outcomes, variances and the appropriateness of care are analysed. This review leads to the identification of improvements in processes and practices with a re-vamped Pathway being drafted which is then implemented in place of the old one, and after another 30–50 cases the outcomes and variances are analysed and reviewed once more; and so continues the cycle. In this way the Pathways of Care system equates to a Continuous Quality Improvement (CQI) system.

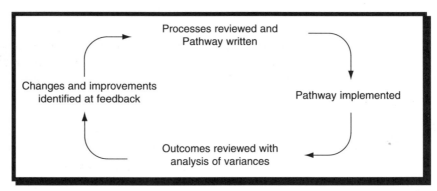

Fig. 1.3 A Pathway quality cycle.

What do Pathways offer?

Pathways of Care offer a health care delivery organisation many valuable benefits relating to the quality and cost of patient care (Fig. 1.4). We shall now consider these in turn.

Benefits from Pathways

(1) Improved patient outcomes
(2) Improved teamwork by caregivers
(3) Improved consistency in care
(4) Increased patient involvement in care
(5) Continuous clinical audit
(6) Clinical and non-clinical resource management
(7) Continuous standard/guideline monitoring
(8) Assistance with risk management
(9) Organisation-wide involvement in a CQI process

Fig. 1.4   Potential benefits to be gained from using Pathways of Care.

Improved patient outcomes

Virginia Bottomley, Secretary of State for Health in 1994, highlighted the importance of 'clinical effectiveness', which she defined as the attainment of good outcomes which improve the quality of the patient's life (Bottomley 1993). Clinical outcomes are of importance in health care, as the NHS has an obligation to ensure that the care it is delivering provides for good outcomes for the patient, which reflects the quality of care that service is providing (Pearson 1987).

However, it is one thing to measure outcomes of care; to improve upon these outcomes, we must do more than simply measure the end result (Johnson 1995). We must also review the current processes and practices of care delivery and link those to the measured outcomes, and then, most importantly, we must review all this data and change, modify and improve those processes and practices in order that the outcomes may also be improved upon.

Pathways co-ordinate the care of all the many disciplines so that all are working towards common goals or outcomes for the patient. Care processes and practices are reviewed, resulting in improvements in how health care is delivered to the patient. With outcome driven care that is centred around the patient, and constant review and improvements in that care, the patient outcomes will be improved.

Patients are the most important people in health care and as such any CQI system must have a positive impact on the quality of both the processes and practices of patient care resulting in improved outcomes.

Improved teamwork by care givers

Pathways of Care are written and developed by the health care professionals. All disciplines should be involved, making up a complete multi-disciplinary team. Simply by getting different disciplines together to discuss and review care processes and practices, the inter-disciplinary barriers may be melted. Staff can better understand the roles of other disciplines and what skills they each have to offer. For example, doctors can find out what an occupational therapist really does; nurses can learn what a speech therapist really has to offer the team; dietitians can find out exactly what a surgical consultant's role entails.

Inter-disciplinary understanding builds up the team so they can work together cohesively and complimentarily; effective patient care requires the skills of all members of the multi-disciplinary team to be working together for the achievement of high quality patient outcomes.

Improved consistency in care

Standardisation of clinical treatments and patient care is a topic that provokes much debate, and 'consistency' of care often gets mixed up in this argument.

Consistency in care is where patients can expect similar, consistent practices and treatments for similar, consistent conditions, whichever practitioner is delivering that care. Any patient attending a hospital for a procedure should be able to expect that the team of doctors, nurses and theatre staff who attend them within that hospital will provide similar, consistent and the best practice for that hospital. Patients should not have to hope to be placed under the care of one consultant's team rather than another, simply because their practices and outcomes are different. Each hospital or organisation should be striving to deliver consistently the best patient care for each condition, no matter which team within that institution is managing the care. Surely this is common sense and what you and I as potential patients have every right to expect? According to Musfeldt & Hart (1993), reducing variation in the process of providing a service is the most effective way of improving quality.

Pathways enable teams to get together and agree practice that is research-based and the best that can be achieved within the resources locally available. Consensus on such 'best practice' that is realistic and achievable is agreed by all the different staff members for each client group. This is laid out, like a guideline, in the Pathway for all to follow. In this way, different processes of care delivery for different teams may be made more consistent through the use of a Pathway.

There are definite links here with standardisation of care. The main argument against standardisation of patient care is that all patients are individuals with their own needs, fears and pathologies. This is true, indeed, and if a Pathway set out a protocol of treatment that was compulsory for all staff to follow, then the individualities of each patient would certainly be ignored. However when you select a patient group whether by diagnosis, condition, procedure or need (e.g. myocardial infarction, endoscopy, uncontrolled pain), there are common threads in terms of what the health care professionals will do for each individual within that group. Such common threads can be mapped out on the Pathway, which is then used as a guideline, with the practitioner using their clinical judgement on whether to follow the anticipated care on the Pathway, or to deviate from that care. Such deviations are recorded as part of the Pathway document, thus providing a facility by which care may be individualised as appropriate. Variance tracking will be considered in depth in Chapters 2 and 3.

Increased patient involvement in care

The Pathway maps out expected care and treatment for specific patient groups or case-types. The Pathway document accompanies the patient throughout their episode of care. Within acute hospital settings the Pathway is usually kept at the patient's bedside, and the document is open to the patient at all times. Indeed, with the best programmes patients are encouraged to read and follow the Pathway throughout their episode of care. At the first contact with the patient, the Pathway is explained by a clinical professional, with the emphasis being made on the Pathway as the *anticipated* plan of care. The Patient Charter (DoH 1992) states that each patient has the right to expect full information on their care and treatment, even prior to their admission to hospital, and Pathways have a significant role to play here.

Once the patient is fully informed of what they can expect, and when things will happen to them, they can then follow their 'map' of care and also participate more in their own care. For instance, if the Pathway states that the patient should drink more than two litres of fluid in 24 hours, the patient can take a more active role in ensuring they achieve this, rather than relying on the nursing staff to repeatedly remind the patient to 'take another drink' every half hour.

The Pathway acts like a map for the patient, letting them know where they are going, what they are likely to come across on their journey, and when their journey through the particular episode is likely to end. In this way, the patient is better informed, and thus more able to participate in their own care.

Continuous audit data

The recording and analysis of variances is covered in detail in Chapters 2 and 3. The analysis of variances provides continuous audit data on the care being delivered. Such audit information is specific for each case-type on the Pathways being analysed, and thus is not discipline-confined, providing genuine clinical audit. The care delivered by the whole multi-disciplinary team for each case-type is thus audited and reviewed with each analysis of the variances. The regular review of care (processes, practices and outcomes) through the analysis of variances and the local team feedback of the data gained, is a vital component of the Pathway tool. Analyses can highlight specific areas that need a more detailed audit, and thus stimulate audit projects; or the Pathway document may be used to collect audit information which is then elicited on analysis. In this way, Pathways of Care are a significant clinical audit tool.

Clinical and non-clinical resource management

Resource management is an important component of quality health care delivery today. The costs of providing good care are rising; high technology treatments now available are an expensive commodity, and more people are surviving previously fatal diseases and living to an old age. The number of cases requiring care and treatment from health care providers is increasing. Economic pressures are high, and all providers need to ensure that resources are well managed, well used and not wasted.

Clinical resources, such as blood tests, X-rays, prostheses, wound dressings and drugs must be managed carefully. Pathways can help to ensure that blood tests, X-rays and electrocardiograph recordings are done when it is clinically appropriate, and so avoid such tests being performed when they are not clinically required or relevant within a specific situation. Every pathology department in all provider units will speak of their raised activity levels in August of each year, when the newly qualified doctors appear on the wards. Because of their inexperience, the junior doctors take many more blood tests than are required, just in case they miss something. These tests are costly to the pathology laboratories and mean patients are needlessly bled in many cases. Pathways for each diagnosis or client group can suggest the appropriate tests to be performed, and in this way provide guidelines for the new doctors to follow.

Equally the Pathway can ensure that the tests required are performed at the appropriate stage of recovery; for example, cardiac enzyme blood tests post-myocardial infarction taken at the optimal time to get the best results, or a hip X-ray taken post-surgery at the specified time for the best result. By guiding the use of clinical resources, even to the extent of suggesting drug prescriptions as agreed by the team for certain case types, Pathways of Care have a major role in clinical resource management.

Non-clinical resources like staff time and equipment must equally be well managed to minimise waste. It is estimated that up to 80% of hospital costs are on staffing, which accounts for millions of pounds each day. Pathways of Care facilitate the co-ordination of patient care delivery, and synchronise the activities performed by all the disciplines involved for each case-type. For example, the occupational therapy staff (OTs) within one orthopaedic unit where I worked stated on a Pathway when they felt was the most appropriate time for them to assess a patient for washing and dressing after a total hip replacement.

Prior to the Pathway being implemented, the OTs were receiving referrals from the ward far too early in the patient's recovery. The OTs within this unit assessed their patients within 24 hours of the referral, and hence in the majority of times that the OT came to see the patient they were still recovering in the immediate post-operative phases and were not in a suitable state to receive the therapy. This meant a wasted visit to the ward, and a return visit would have to be arranged a few days later. This waste of time has been dramatically improved upon since the OTs have set out on the Pathway which post-operative day the referral is to be sent to their department. Now the number of inappropriate referrals and wasted ward visits has dropped significantly, enabling the therapists to make better, more effective use of their time.

Staff time spent on documentation is an increasing problem, particularly in the high throughput areas such as day surgery. Pathways of Care can help to provide integrated non-duplicative paperwork that is quick to use for all disciplines and this facility is of particular relevance to high volume day care units.

Many Pathway programmes within the UK have now reported reductions in lengths of stay, and in these ways, Pathways of Care have a significant effect on non-clinical resource management too through better bed utilisation.

Continuous standard and guideline monitoring

For many years, standardised treatment regimes, practice guidelines and protocols have been developed through the Royal Colleges and professional bodies, in an effort to set minimum standards and to promote consistent best practice. Practice guidelines have been defined as:

'Systematically developed statements to assist practitioner and patient decisions about appropriate healthcare for specific clinical circumstances.'

(Institute of Medicine 1992)

A guideline is simply a guide to assist decisions about appropriate health care. A useful description of guidelines is taken from the bulletin on *Effective Health Care* (1994):

'Guidelines should identify recommendations for appropriate and cost effective management of clinical conditions or the appropriate use of clinical procedures with the principal aim of promoting good performance'.

In this way, a Pathway of Care is a guideline, in that a Pathway sets out recommendations for appropriate care and treatments, as agreed by the local multi-disciplinary team, whilst facilitating good practices. We have already discussed how Pathways can contribute to the management of resources and the provision of consistent practice, and in a similar manner the development of guidelines to rationalise the use of investigations, tests and treatments is now widely recommended. Therefore it can be seen that Pathways are effectively locally determined guidelines for practice.

Guidelines are more likely to be effective if they take into account local circumstances, are disseminated throughout an organisation by an active educational programme, and are integrated into the common records used by staff in everyday practice situations. These issues are just as pertinent for Pathways; they must consider local circumstances when written, to reflect local best practice, and the Pathway document must be made part of the patient record and used as such by all disciplines so that the Pathway may act as a specific reminder directly relating to professional activity at the patient bedside.

Many national guidelines are now being written by the Royal Colleges and professional bodies, for example British Thoracic Society Guidelines for Care of the Asthmatic Patient, National Clinical Guideline for the Prevention and Management of Pressure Sores, etc. Health care provider organisations also have many locally written guidelines (e.g. local guidelines for the management of anticoagulant therapy, local guidelines for the assessment of pain control, etc.). National or local guidelines can be incorporated into a Pathway, which will provide the means to ensure that the guidelines are used by professionals to inform their decisions regarding care and treatment. Throughout the world, clinical guidelines are being promoted as a means to improve practices and in turn, the quality of patient care. However, simply writing a guideline does not ensure that it is then used in practice. Pathways offer a tool for the successful implementation and integration of guidelines into real clinical practice.

Pathways also provide a locally owned facility by which clinical teams can monitor their activities against the practice guidelines. With a guideline set out in the Pathway, any detour from that Pathway which is documented as a variance can demonstrate where the guideline is not being followed, with a reason for that deviation also being documented.

A standard is defined as: 'Professionally developed expressions of the range of acceptable variation from a norm or criterion' (Donabedian 1982). Standards are being written by all provider units, and by all disciplines, yet simply writing such standards does nothing to improve the quality of care provision. The institution also needs to monitor its current level of achievement against the set standards, to highlight areas in need of improvement.

Such standards can also be monitored through Pathways. For example, if a pharmacy department sets a turn-around time standard of three hours for the processing of 'to take away' drugs (TTAs), this can be monitored on the Pathway by adding a box to fill in the time the TTA prescription chart left the ward, and another box to fill in when the TTAs arrived on the ward. This time lapse can then be measured and monitored to see what percentage of cases are not adhering to the set standard. In the same way Patient Charter Standards may be measured using Pathways.

In this way Pathways of Care can be used to monitor adherence to guidelines and the achievement of agreed standards.

Assistance with risk management

Chapter 13 explains the role Pathways play in risk management. Pathways offer the clinical team the opportunity to anticipate risk, and to instigate strategies to prevent unwanted situations arising by reviewing potential risks when constructing the Pathways. Pathways of Care also provide a care delivery setting which is considered, and regularly reviewed; such a controlled setting is less prone to claims of negligence (see Chapter 12, Pathways of Care, Clinical Guidelines and the Law).

Organisation-wide involvement in a CQI process

For a Continuous Quality Improvement (CQI) process to be effective in improving the quality of patient care, it is essential for all staff to be involved. A patient may be seen by more than 40 different members of staff within one hospital admission, from domestic to doctor. All these staff members must know about, understand and be involved in any CQI process that will result in an improved patient experience. An organisation-wide Pathway programme will keep all involved staff informed of what is required by them in the delivery of health care, and a successful programme will feed back all the results of analyses of care to all disciplines so they can see how they are performing against expected guidelines and standards, and can also see the benefits and improvements being achieved by the teams.

Conclusion

As an introduction, this chapter has set out an overview of what Pathways of Care have to offer health care provider units. Pathways provide a proactive locally owned facility by which clinical teams can review and improve their processes and practices of care delivery towards the achievement of agreed clinical outcomes through the provision of best local practice. Pathways also offer a tool to aid with clinical and non-clinical resource management, risk management and the provision of more information for patients, set within the broad context of clinical audit. Such a tool cannot be overlooked by health care providers in today's health care system.

References

Bottomley, V. (1993) Priority setting in the NHS. In *Rationing in Action*. BMJ Publishing Group, London.

Department of Health (1992) *The Patient's Charter*. HMSO, London.

Donabedian, A. (1982) *The Criteria of Standards of Quality*, 2, 9. Health Administration Press, Michigan.

Effective Health Care bulletin (1994) Implementing clinical practice guidelines; can guidelines be used to improve clinical practices?. December. University of Leeds.

Institute of Medicine (1992) *Guidelines for Clinical Practice; from Development to Use* (eds M.J. Field & K.N. Lohr). National Academy Press, Washington DC.

Johnson, S. (1995) Pathways to the heart of care quality. *Nursing Management*, 1(8) January, 26–7.

Musfeldt, C. & Hart, R.I. (1993) Physician-directed diagnostic and therapeutic plans; a quality cure for America's health-care crisis. *Journal of the Society for Health Systems*, 4(1) 80–87.

Pearson, A. (1987) Outcome measures. In *Nursing Quality Measurement* (ed. A. Pearson) John Wiley & Sons, London.

Chapter 2

What is a Pathway of Care?

Sue Johnson

Introduction

Chapter 1 gave an overall introduction to Pathways of Care, with explanations of the potential benefits that may be gained from their use for the patient, care workers and health care organisations. This chapter will answer the question 'What is a Pathway of Care ?'.

Within the context of health care delivery there are many different clinical settings, from community and mental health to acute care. Each of these settings has its own unique requirements and demands in terms of information and workload. Any method of organising care delivery and upgrading the corresponding documentation must be driven by the unique needs of each setting. Therefore any model of care management cannot be uniformly applied across the board; it must be adaptable to the chosen setting. Thus Pathways will be discussed as a concept or generalised tool within this chapter, with Part 2 of the book demonstrating the ways in which the tool has been applied in various clinical settings.

A Pathway involves all members of the multi-disciplinary team, from the development and construction of the Pathway to its analysis and the feedback of results. A Pathway that is unidisciplinary limits its potential for the audit and improvement of care.

What is a Pathway of Care?

A useful analogy to explain the concept of Pathways is that of a hat shop. Many different customers come to that shop, all having their own individual heads; some heads are wide, some thin, some have big ears, some have small ears, some heads have thick hair on them, and some are bald. All the heads are different and individual to each customer. When the customer enters the hat shop they will have in mind the type or design of hat they wish to purchase, with their choice being individual to them, from straw boaters to bowler hats. Therefore when they come into the shop each customer, irrespective of their own individualities, has a common generalised goal: that of purchasing a hat.

Once in the shop, the shop assistant will go through the same motions and processes of activities with each different customer. They will measure and size up the customer's head, help them to find the design of hat they require, and assist them in trying the hats on until the customer chooses the hat they want. The shop assistant then takes the customer to the cash desk to wrap up the hat and exchange it for payment. The customer then leaves the hat shop fully satisfied with the service they have received. Notice that all the different customers want the same generalised outcome from their visit to the shop – that of buying a hat that fits and is of the design they wish – and the process that the shop assistant goes through is common for each customer for the realisation of the desired common goal.

In the same way, for select groups of patients or clients common goals and outcomes of care may be determined, and the processes of care delivery from all the care workers involved will also be similar, in spite of the individualities of each of the different patients, due to the general common goals that are being strived for.

Pathways of Care are a concept, a generalised idea. A definition of Pathways of Care is:

> 'Pathways of Care amalgamate all the anticipated elements of care and treatment of all members of the multi-disciplinary team, for a patient or client of a particular case-type or grouping within an agreed time frame, for the achievement of agreed outcomes. Any deviation from the plan is documented as a "variance"; the analysis of which provides information for the review of current practice'.

When the concept of Pathways is made manifest, they may be used as a tool in two major areas: a clinical management tool and a clinical audit tool (Fig. 2.1).

Clinical management tool

Select case-type or client group

The first stage for the development of a Pathway is the selection of a client group or case-type. There are many ways to select a grouping of cases, and the method used will depend on the clinical setting. Groupings may be made based on diagnosis, procedure performed, patient need or even stage of treatment. Within the acute setting diagnostic or procedural groupings

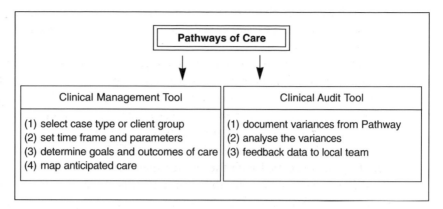

Fig. 2.1   Elements of the Pathway tool.

are commonly used, whilst in the community or long-term settings patient need or stage of treatment may be used (Fig. 2.2).

Selecting a case-type or grouping is important, as it dictates the difficulty or ease with which the Pathway can be constructed. The more defined the grouping, the simpler it is to set time frames, and map out care; the more unspecified the grouping the harder it is to map expected activities and care. It is worth choosing a grouping that is well-defined for the early Pathways

Diagnosis:	e.g.	Myocardial infarction
		Deep vein thrombosis
		Cerebrovascular accident
		Subdural haemorrhage
Procedure:	e.g.	Circumcision
		Total knee replacement
		Hernia repair
		Abdominal hysterectomy
		Endoscopy
		Arthroscopy
		Induction of labour
Patient need:	e.g.	Uncontrolled pain
		Incontinence
		Inability to read due to loss of sight
		Lack of understanding of diabetes
Stage/phase of treatment:	e.g.	Initial assessment
		Discharge preparation
		Post-discharge phase

Fig. 2.2   Client or case-type groupings.

piloted within an organisation, to make the process of developing the pilot Pathway documents easier for the clinical teams involved.

For example, a broad grouping of asthmatics for a proposed Pathway will be difficult to develop; paediatric asthmatics require different interventions of care and treatments from adult asthmatics. Equally many asthmatics who present at hospital with an asthmatic attack have an associated chest infection. Should the proposed Pathway include asthmatics who have a chest infection, or will it be only for those presenting with an attack not related to a chest infection? Within the grouping of 'asthmatic' there are many sub-groupings which could each have a different Pathway for treatment. Thought must be put into selecting the group of clients for whom the Pathway will be designed. It may be more appropriate to select a specified group of 'asthmatic children under 16 years of age, presenting with asthmatic attack, not associated with a chest infection'. Selection of the grouping must be determined by the local team, who have a working knowledge of what types of cases present themselves to their particular setting (Table 2.1).

Table 2.1   Select a client group.

Client group/case-type: adult acute myocardial infarction

Set time frame and parameters

Once the case-type or client group is selected, a time frame must be set. The time frame provides the parameters for the Pathway: the point at which the particular Pathway will commence and the point at which it will finish; for example, a Pathway for a selected group of myocardial infarction (MI) patients could start and finish at a variety of intervals. It could commence when the patient arrives in the accident and emergency department, or it could start with the ambulance teams when they arrive at the patient's home. Equally it could end at the point of discharge from hospital, or be completed when the patient has finished cardiac rehabilitation classes and attended the six month post-MI outpatient follow-up appointment. The team needs to be clear upon what point the chosen Pathway is to start and finish (Fig. 2.3).

A time frame is also required for the arrangement of care within the parameters previously set. Care can be arranged or mapped out on a day by day basis – which may be appropriate for surgical situations – or on an hour by hour basis, which could be used within an emergency setting. Equally, care could be mapped out within phases or stages which do not in themselves have a fixed amount of time attached. For example, within mental health it may be more appropriate for care to be set out in phases or stages,

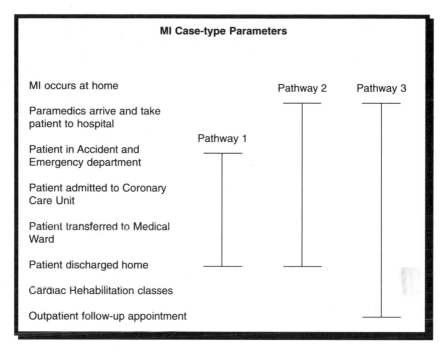

Fig. 2.3 Setting the parameters for a Pathway.

that do not relate to fixed periods of time, depending on the progress of the client for whom that Pathway was constructed.

The whole team involved in constructing the Pathway must be involved in deciding the method for the division of care within the parameters agreed (Table 2.2).

Determine goals and outcomes of care

With the chosen group of clients and the time frames selected, the team must then decide what the outcomes or goals of care within the chosen parameters will be. Such outcomes may be for the patient to achieve, for staff to achieve on behalf of the patient, or may be process outcomes that must be achieved. For example, the episode of care chosen may have clinical goals for the patient to achieve (e.g. the patient will be able to transfer independently from bed to chair before discharge from hospital, which will require certain interventions from the nursing and therapy staff throughout the episode), or clinical goals for the treatments to achieve (e.g. pain will be well-controlled each day). Process outcomes or goals could be used for administrative procedures (e.g. a referral to physiotherapy for outpatient treatment will be responded to within 48 hours of being received).

Table 2.2   Division of care stages within parameters for the selected client group.

Client group/case-type:	adult acute myocardial infarction
Parameters:	from arrival in accident and emergency department to discharge from hospital
Time divisions:	hour by hour in accident and emergency department day by day in ward setting

1st hour in A/E	2nd hour in A/E	day 1 in CCU	day 2 transfer to ward	day 3 ward	day 4 ward	day 5 ward	day 6 discharge home

Determining the goals for the end of the chosen episode of care enables the multi-disciplinary team to direct care provision towards the common goals, each working together in the same direction. At the same time, goals of care may be set for each day or each stage of the Pathway. The achievement of these goals and outcomes may then be monitored when the Pathways are analysed, with the reasons for the goals not being achieved being recorded too (Table 2.3).

Map anticipated care of all disciplines

With the client group chosen, the time frames determined and the outcomes and goals of care agreed upon, the team can then map out the anticipated activities, interventions, assessments and actions of all disciplines. In order that care may be mapped in this way, current practices and processes of care delivery of the whole multi-disciplinary team need to be reviewed, so the team can understand and identify where actions or assessments are duplicated and how the different professionals interact. Armed with this information, the expected care is set out for each day or phase of the Pathway (Table 2.4).

Clinical audit tool

Document variances from anticipated Pathway

Inherent to Pathways of Care is the facility of 'variance'. A 'variance' is defined as any deviation from the expected care identified on the Pathway.

Table 2.3 Setting the goals of care.

Client group/case-type:	adult acute myocardial infarction
Parameters:	from arrival in accident and emergency department to discharge from hospital
Time divisions:	hour by hour in accident and emergency department day by day in ward setting
goals for care: within 24 hours:	diagnosis obtained thrombolysis administered within 30 mins chest pain controlled admitted to coronary care unit
within 72 hours:	information on MI given to patient patient understands information on MI seen by dietitian seen by cardiac counsellor
within 6 days:	no chest pain no signs of secondary heart failure outpatient appointment booked criteria for discharge met mobilising fully without chest pain

This facility is an essential component of the Pathway tool, as without the inbuilt ability for the clinical professional to vary the planned treatments according to the individual needs of the patient or client, the care for that patient or client cannot be individualised. The Pathway would then become a checklist of interventions to be followed, and would not allow for clinical judgement in determining whether or not the care planned was appropriate. A Pathway tool without the variance facility would create a 'cook-book medicine' approach to care delivery.

Any detour from the anticipated Pathway is recorded on the Pathway document as a 'variance'. A variance tracking sheet is used for the documentation of variances. A variance may be recorded due to a planned intervention not being performed as written on the anticipated Pathway, or due to an extra intervention or activity being performed that was not written on the Pathway (Fig. 2.4).

When variances are recorded, the date of the variance taking place, the reasons for that variance and the action that was taken as a result of that variance are all written down. Recording of variances should be performed by all disciplines, with each individual variance being recorded

Table 2.4   Mapping care within time frames, for all disciplines.

1st hour in A/E	2nd hour in A/E	CCU day 1	day 2	day 3
baseline TPR and BP ECG medical assessment thrombolysis cardiac monitor bedrest	refer to on-call team refer to CCU transfer to CCU cardiac monitor half hourly BP and P family informed bedrest	cardiac monitor 2 hourly TPR and BP full medical clerking nursing assessment refer cardiac counsellor refer dietitian bedrest	transfer to ward mobile around bed monitor discontinued 4 hourly TPR and BP independent hygiene information leaflets	4 hourly TPR and BP mobile to toilet independent hygiene discuss information seen by counsellor seen by dietitian discharge date set

Date	Variance and reason for it	Action taken
1 January	Patient not discharged as not able to transfer from bed to chair independently	Patient and family informed of decision, with reasons explained. Doctor to review situation with team in two days
3 March	Intravenous infusion not discontinued as patient not tolerating oral fluids	Doctor prescribed more IV fluids, and to review patient in morning. Patient to continue with sips of fluid today.
18 June	Full social assessment not performed by social worker as patient not co-operating	Key worker informed, and social worker to talk with family tomorrow to gain information on social circumstances

Fig. 2.4   Example of variance tracking.

by the clinical professional who was involved with that variance taking place.

A variance is not a failure in care. A variance simply records a change to the expected or planned care on the Pathway as is appropriate for the individual patient at that particular point in time. In this way clinical autonomy and professional judgement can be maintained in deciding what is the correct and best care for their patient.

Analyse the variances

Once the variances from the expected care are recorded, they are reviewed or analysed at regular intervals, thereby providing a clinical audit tool. The Pathway sets out the expected care, which can be equated with a common line or guideline of care; the variances are effectively any detour off this common line on either side. Analysis of these variances compared with the common line or guideline provides audit data on what is taking place, and what goals or outcomes are being achieved.

Feedback data to team

Analysing the variances is of no use unless the information gained is fed back to the local team for consideration. The team can then review what is currently taking place, and upgrade the Pathway with agreed changes to the document resulting from improvements in practices and processes of care

Patient condition:	pyrexia
	chest pain
	dehydration
	pain not controlled
	incontinent
	wound infected
	communication difficulties
	hard of hearing
	confused
Staff or people:	nurse decision
	nurse not available
	doctor decision
	doctor not available
	physiotherapy decision
	speech therapist not available
	patient decision
	family not available
System:	equipment not available
	department closed (weekend or holiday)
	theatres running late
	operation cancelled
Community:	social services not available
	transport delay
	nursing home placement delay

Fig. 2.5 Examples of variance code groupings.

delivery. In this way true clinical audit is performed, with the closure of the audit loop through changes and improvements in care.

The analysis of variances can become a time consuming and extensive exercise when there are many Pathways to review. Many sites code the variances to aid analysis. For example, variances may be coded by 'patient condition', 'staff or people', 'system', and other groupings. Figure 2.5 gives samples of these coding groupings, with examples of the type of variances allocated to each grouping. Each of these anticipated variances is then allocated a number, which then facilitates automated methods of analysis; this is relevant when there is a large quantity of Pathways to analyse.

Conclusion

Pathways of Care are a simple concept and a useful tool that enable a clinical team to manage and audit its care for the patient. The tool sets out the core elements of care and treatment of all members of the multi-disciplinary team for a patient or client of a particular case-type or grouping, for the achievement of agreed outcomes. Any deviation from the plan is documented as a variance; the analysis of which provides information for the review of current practice.

Chapter 3

Analysis of Variation from the Pathway

Denise Kitchiner

'... you don't have to know what you are doing in order to do what you are doing'

(Keillor 1994)

Introduction

Pathways set the standards of care for a patient with a particular condition in a specific hospital or community setting. They define the care which the patient should receive, together with the expected progress for that condition, within a specified timescale (Coffey *et al*. 1992). An essential part of the use of Pathways is collecting and analysing the information obtained when a patient deviates from the Pathway. A 'variance' is defined as any deviation from what was expected to happen.

Why is variation from the Pathway important?

Analysis of the variation provides accurate information on the frequency and the cause of variations in patient care. The analysis encourages members of the multi-disciplinary team to adhere to the guidelines and standards set in the Pathway, or justify the reason for the variation. This improves clinical outcomes and the quality of patient care by reducing avoidable variation in the clinical process (Hart & Musfeldt 1992; James 1993; Weilitz & Potter 1993). Analysis of variation from the Pathway is a powerful audit tool as all aspects of patient care are constantly reviewed and revised. Improvements in the quality of care are rapidly achieved by continuously re-defining the Pathways to reflect current best practice. This facilitates the inclusion of multi-disciplinary audit and continuous quality improvement into routine clinical practice. Early in the development and use of Pathways, it is important to establish a formal mechanism for collecting and analysing information about variations from the Pathway and their causes.

A term commonly used to describe the analysis of variation from the Pathway is 'variance analysis'. However this term has a specific meaning in statistical terminology (Kendall *et al*. 1983), so it is preferable to use the term 'analysis of variation from the Pathway', so as not to confuse the process with the more statistical term.

When analysing deviation from the expected, it is important to have accurate information on the normal course of events for that particular condition. Therefore when designing a Pathway it is essential to base the Pathway on what actually happens. This data may be obtained by reviewing the experiences of patients recently treated for the same condition, or by consultation with the multi-disciplinary team to develop a Pathway which accurately represents current patient care and progress in that particular institution. This should include the length of stay, and identify days or times at which specific activities are carried out. National guidelines (Thomson *et al*. 1995) and evidence-based research (Rosenberg & Donald 1995) can also be incorporated into the Pathway. This information must also be constantly updated (Thomson *et al*. 1995). As data is collected from patients managed on the Pathway, this is added to the body of information available about that condition and the 'expected' course of events will change accordingly.

The aims of analysis of variation

The aims of analysis of variation can be summarised as follows:

(1) To determine the variation from the goals of treatment
(2) To determine the cause of variation
(3) To find solutions to avoidable delays
(4) To investigate and analyse specific problems identified
(5) To redefine the Pathway in the light of the most recent experience

Determining variation from the goals of treatment

In order to determine variation from goals, the goals must first be defined. A Pathway is divided into time intervals during which specific goals and expected progress are defined, together with investigations and treatment. There are usually between one and five important goals in each time interval of a Pathway, which must be achieved for a patient to progress towards a timely discharge or completion of treatment. Goals are most commonly specified on a daily basis, yet hourly goals may be more appropriate in emergency care, such as with major trauma. Weekly goals may be indicated in the management of a chronic condition. As an example, consider a patient admitted for elective surgery; important goals must be achieved before the operation can take place. On the day of operation the patient must be suitably starved before surgery, and after the operation the intravenous infusion needs to be discontinued when the patient is able to tolerate oral fluids. Such goals need to be achieved in order that the patient achieves recovery and discharge without unnecessary delay. It is essential to identify the goals which are important in each particular set of circumstances and to collect all the necessary information on these.

When deciding which goals or variables to analyse, there are points to bear in mind. Goals which improve patient care and efficiency of treatment should be given a high priority. Data should always include the clinical outcome of the treatment given. Goals which improve the cost-effectiveness of the care provided should also be considered. The development of a Pathway may reveal an area where evidence-based information regarding the best method of treatment does not exist (Rosenberg & Donald 1995). This may stimulate a research project to gather the necessary information. Design of the Pathway can facilitate collection of data, and analysis of variation may provide the results of the research question raised. Improved patient care can then be facilitated by redefining the Pathway to incorporate the results of research.

For analysis one should choose goals where variations have been identified or are likely to occur. Some key interventions may take place so consistently that there is no need to analyse them; for example, it is essential to have blood products available for patients undergoing major surgery. If this is always done efficiently there is no need to analyse this aspect of care. If however, operations have been delayed as these products are not always made available, this would be an important goal to analyse in order to identify the causes of inefficiencies. Although some data collected will be the same for all clinical conditions within the same department or directorate, some will vary for different conditions. Entirely different goals may be appropriate for each condition, particularly if the care given and outcomes expected are different.

Criteria for choosing the variables will also vary, depending on priorities in individual institutions or particular problems which have been locally identified. For these reasons goals or variables are usually unique for a particular institution, even for patients with the same condition. The variables being analysed will also change with time. If a problem which was causing variation is resolved and this aspect of care is then performed consistently well, there may be no need to continue analysing it. This allows time to be spent on resolving the causes of avoidable variations in another aspect of patient care. The goals to be analysed will be identified by members of the multi-disciplinary team from examination of variations from the Pathways, or may be influenced by outside parties such as the purchasers of health care, community workers or patients themselves. These may include the length of stay in hospital or in the intensive care unit, specific information to be given to patients or community health workers on discharge, or details regarding investigations and treatment.

Determining the causes of variation

When determining the causes of a variation, it is important to know whether it was avoidable or unavoidable. An unavoidable variance is one over which the health care team and the patient have no control; for example, a patient who develops an infection the day before an operation will have his operation cancelled and this is unavoidable. But this situation requires further evaluation; if the patient's blood count showed a markedly raised white cell count at the pre-admission clinic the week prior to admission, and the result of this test was only reviewed on the night before surgery, then the resulting loss of an operation session due to the lateness of cancellation preventing a re-booking of the theatre time for another case, could have been potentially avoided.

It is usually unnecessary to concentrate time and effort on analysing unavoidable variances. An exception to this may be those variations which take the form of complications which require further evaluation. If unavoidable variances occur frequently, they must be examined to ensure that there is no underlying avoidable problem. For example, if a piece of equipment breaks down once or twice, this may be unavoidable; yet if this situation occurs frequently, the reliability of the piece of equipment must be questioned and a solution to the problem found. By documenting all variances, this type of problem may be highlighted.

Some causes of variation are potentially avoidable. These are ones when something can be done to reduce the occurrence or the frequency of that particular variation. These variances require more detailed information for the analysis in order that improvements can be planned and implemented. In some cases it may be difficult to determine whether a problem or delay was entirely unavoidable. For example, a patient who has post-operative complications may spend extra days in the intensive care unit and this is unavoidable. However, further delay can occur when the patient is fit for transfer to a general ward and there are no beds available on the ward. With such variations it is necessary to classify variance into avoidable, unavoidable or a combination of both (Fig. 3.1).

```
                    Variance classification
  • avoidable
  • unavoidable
  • combination
```

Fig. 3.1 Classification of types of variance.

Variation can further be broken down into five important groups, depending on the precise cause of that variation (Fig. 3.2). Patients may deviate from the Pathway because they have a more severe illness than most others with the same condition; a family may cause variation because they do not agree to a recommended course of treatment; medical staff can cause avoidable delays in discharging a patient if all the required investigations are not completed on time, or if they do not have enough time to complete the tasks necessary for the patient's progress towards discharge; the system may cause delay through a lack or a failure in equipment or a lack of support staff; community services may be the cause of a delay in discharge preparations due to the inability to find an appropriate placement for the patient on discharge.

```
                    Variance groupings
  • patient condition
  • family
  • clinical staff
  • system
  • community
```

Fig. 3.2 Groupings of variances.

In order to obtain accurate data on the cause of variation, further information may be needed. For example, if an avoidable variation is occurring commonly, such as a lack of nursing staff within the theatres, this system cause of a variation, once identified, may be analysed separately and in more depth until a solution is found.

Finding solutions to avoidable variations

Having identified the causes of the most important avoidable variations, the next task is to find solutions to these problems. Some variations need very little planning to find the appropriate solution. Others require the introduction of fairly simple measures to overcome and prevent the situation recurring in the future. Yet others will only be solved by long-term planning and co-operation of a number of health care professionals, often in conjunction with the managers.

Rapid response to avoidable variation is often done automatically, when staff caring for the patients take action immediately to solve potential variations. Pathways highlight variances and encourage staff to make an early and appropriate response, thereby preventing delays in progress for the patient. There are a number of advantages to having this information on the variance tracking or analysis sheet. It focuses on responsibility and makes staff evaluate whether or not what they are doing is appropriate for their patient.

The action taken as a result of a variance may be important from a medico-legal viewpoint, and it is important that such actions are clearly documented at the time. In addition, valuable information can be obtained by evaluating and analysing the actions taken when a variance is documented. Was the action appropriate to the circumstances? Did the action result in a permanent resolution of the problem or did the variance or problem recur when other staff were faced with the same situation? Was information regarding the variance passed on to the correct people? Was the patient informed of the cause of the variance and what was being done about it; was the patient reassured with this explanation?

Such information often indicates the most appropriate method of resolving any problem. It also involves all members of the multi-disciplinary team in finding solutions to an avoidable variance. If this proactive approach to patient care is used, there is a great advantage in having someone to review the patients on a daily basis so that avoidable variations to the expected care can rapidly be detected and acted upon. However, this is labour-intensive and when many patients are treated in accordance with a Pathway, this may well be extremely impractical.

Analysis of avoidable variations will indicate areas where there are consistent inefficiencies. It will indicate the frequency and the causes, and may even provide the solutions to the problems. Often small changes in practice can result in a much more efficient system. In particular, understanding the role of other members of the multi-disciplinary team will result in better communication and co-operation, leading to an improved performance by the team. Data allows staff to modify inappropriate practice and confirms the benefits of current practice in a quantifiable manner.

Some variances need careful planning to overcome. It is sometimes necessary to involve other disciplines such as management, therapists, ancillary staff, community workers or general practitioners, in solving the problems. Information obtained from analysis provides the necessary data as a starting point to indicate which members of the team need to be involved. Analysis of the causes of variation informs the decisions regarding solutions to the problems identified.

Analysis allows acceptable solutions to be found more easily; locally collected information is credible, non-threatening and relevant to that local team. Improvements are more likely to be accomplished if the information is owned by the staff involved in patient care. Solutions are more likely to be accepted by the local staff if all members of the local team are instrumental in finding the solutions and implementing the agreed changes. Management also has a commitment in this regard. If the inefficiencies are caused by problems in the system, the managers must help address these problems. However, it is much easier to get the co-operation of managers in this if facts and figures are available from the analyses.

Investigating and analysing specific problems

Sometimes development of a Pathway or analysis of the variations indicates that there is a problem that requires more detailed information to be collated in order that a solution may be found. The Pathways provide the opportunity to collect and then analyse such additional information as the Pathway can be redesigned to collect the necessary information, or an audit project may be set up to look at a specific aspect of care in much more detail.

Equally, various methods of treatment can be compared when using Pathways. If two health professionals cannot agree on a standard method of patient care management, a Pathway can be developed for each of the two methods. Once the Pathways are used, the outcomes of each method can then be compared; if there is no significant difference in the outcomes of each method of patient management, then the teams may choose the simplest or more cost-effective method of treatment.

Redefining Pathways to reflect best current practice

The last, but not the least important aim of analysis of variation, is to redefine the Pathway. A Pathway is a dynamic document based on an ongoing evaluation of care. It is important to ensure that the Pathway represents current practice and not what was being done two or three years before. Without the feedback of results, analysis of variation from the Pathway cannot produce the necessary benefits. Improvements in care, together with any specific recommendations or guidelines, can be rapidly incorporated into current practice by redefining the Pathways accordingly. This results in continuous improvement in the quality of care provided.

What should be analysed?

When considering analysis of variation, it is important to realise that Pathways fall into two groups. Some Pathways are very simple and all the data which is collected on the Pathway can be analysed; some Pathways contain large amounts of additional data such as the nursing care plan and indications for planned investigations and treatments. It may not then be appropriate, and is usually unproductive, to routinely analyse variation from every detail of care on this type of Pathway. Enough information must be collected and analysed to accurately represent the treatment the patients have received and the causes of important variations in care. However, if large amounts of non-essential data are collected, the more important information may be lost. In general, it is more useful to have detailed information on aspects of care where changes are needed.

Process of analysis

How to record variance

There are a number of different ways in which variances from the Pathway can be recorded. They can be documented directly onto the Pathway, or onto a variance tracking or analysis sheet attached to the Pathway plan.

These sheets should be designed in such a way as to be easy to use, with sufficient space for documentation of the information required; the variance, the cause of that variance and the action taken (Fig. 3.3). The person responsible, of whichever discipline, for any task which does not take place as planned on the Pathway should document this. Any variation from the Pathway should be documented. Identification of a variance is useful in routine patient care, allowing staff to highlight the specific needs of each patient, thereby individualising patient care.

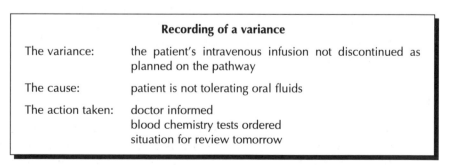

Recording of a variance	
The variance:	the patient's intravenous infusion not discontinued as planned on the pathway
The cause:	patient is not tolerating oral fluids
The action taken:	doctor informed blood chemistry tests ordered situation for review tomorrow

Fig. 3.3   Example of a variance recording.

Variance can be positive or negative. A positive variance occurs when goals are achieved earlier than expected. If such a variance forms a trend, then the Pathway needs to be changed to accommodate it. For example, if the median length of stay of a group of patients on a Pathway is six days, with some patients going home on the fifth day, then as this positive variance becomes the more common experience for each cohort of patients, the Pathway must be changed to accommodate the new common experience. Some centres will actively try to obtain positive variance on every patient (Turley *et al.* 1994), and this proactive approach to Pathways can drive the changes and improvements in the quality and efficiency of patient care. To do this it is necessary to have a case manager role to review the patients regularly and anticipate problems, whilst recognising the opportunities to accelerate recovery for the patient. This proactive approach is probably more suitable for high risk, low volume case types where the care delivered can have an impact on outcome and cost.

How many to analyse?

The written Pathway should, if possible, be stored on a computer system which allows changes to be made quickly and easily. Pathways should be based on recent experience or that of the last thirty patients treated for the same condition. As more recent information becomes available, the data on patients treated earlier should not be included in the Pathway unless there is a good reason to do so.

Common practice in the UK is to analyse approximately 30 cases for each cohort, although this is dependent on the volume of throughput for the specified cases. Many sites now perform analyses at particular time intervals, for instance every six months.

Methods of data collection, entry, analysis and the type of database used will vary considerably between institutions. These differences will reflect traditional practice and the skills and interests of individual members of the multi-disciplinary team. The role of clinical audit is also closely involved in the collection and processing of data from the Pathways, and the methods of analysis will largely depend on the facilities available within the audit department.

Data collection

The data collected is that which is documented on the variance tracking or analysis sheet, the important information being the avoidable variations from the expected Pathway. It is essential to collect some data from all patients whether there has been a variance or not, as such information enables the median experience to be calculated; for instance, length of stay may be collated for all patients and then the median length of stay for the whole cohort can be calculated to ensure that the Pathway still reflects local common practice and activities.

If the Pathway is simple, it will be quite easy to transfer information that is to be analysed directly onto a database for analysis. However, many Pathways contain a large amount of data, much of which will not be required for an analysis. It is important to indicate on the Pathway which information is to be analysed, to encourage staff to complete this section of the Pathway document. If the information on the Pathway is incomplete, the team analysing the Pathways will need to refer back to the patient's notes or other paperwork, which is time consuming and unnecessary. If the required information is not collected from the Pathway, the analysis will be less accurate. Some thought must go into the design of the Pathway document and the variance recording sheets to ensure accurate and full recordings of variances and other important information.

Databases for the analysis of information and data entry

Once information on variances from the expected Pathway is collected from the analysis sheets, it must be transferred onto a database for analysis. Most hospitals within the UK use computerised databases and statistical packages from commercial sources. The choice of a database is an individual one, although there are a number of factors to bear in mind; the package should be easy to use for all staff members; it should be able to perform the kind of analyses you want, collate the information you require and be easily accessible to all disciplines involved in the Pathway process too. Computerised databases are powerful tools (see Chapter 15, Automation of Pathways).

The information that is collected needs to be prepared in a way that facilitates simple transfer to the database, saving time and reducing the potential for errors of transfer. Such data may come from a number of sources:

- Data can be transferred directly from the Pathway or variance tracking sheet onto the database (this is appropriate when most or all the information from a Pathway is to be analysed).
- Data may be initially entered into an information collection summary sheet which has a format similar to the database itself (this can be used when much of the information collected is not required for analysis).
- Data can be coded on the variance tracking sheet and then transferred to the database in a coded format. In this case, the codes must be unam-

biguous as there is more potential for inaccuracy of transfer as coded data is more difficult to recognise.

Only the data to be analysed should be entered onto the database. Entry of large amounts of information which will never be used is unproductive. What information is collected and transferred into the database depends on the local needs of the individual institution or hospital. In general, information commonly entered and analysed include:

- Basic demographic data
- Other clinical conditions or co-morbidities that may influence outcome
- Data on each goal and the variances from those goals
- The reason for each variance occurring
- Clinical outcomes, complications, re-admissions

Collating the reasons for variances occurring is of utmost importance, so the team can elicit whether or not the variation was avoidable and what caused the variance – the family, patient, staff, system or the community.

Data analysis

Data analysis is a skill which may need to be taught, but despite this it is ideally performed by the health professionals using the Pathway; a statistician is not closely involved with the Pathway and hence may not obtain the most appropriate information, nor interpret the findings accurately or in context. Equally, one could argue that an independent statistician or data input worker may be less biased and take the information at face value, without influencing the analyses performed and the conclusions made.

Pathways specify not only what must be done but when it should take place and how often. Therefore many of the events which take place are based on numbers, such as the number of days in hospital or the number of investigations performed. The Pathway reflects the median or mean average of these numbers based on the common experiences of other patients with the same condition. There is a difference between the median and the mean; the mean is the sum of a group of numbers divided by the total number of figures. For example, if a group of patients spend 3, 3, 4, 5 and 30 days in hospital, the mean length of stay is 9 days (45 days divided by 5). The median length of stay is the middle number, so for this cohort of five cases, the median would be 4 days.

The mean value does not accurately reflect the length of stay that one could expect for this type of patient, as it is distorted by the one patient who stayed in for 30 days. The median value, however, gives a more accurate representation of the experience, particularly when there is wide variation in the numbers being analysed. Thus it is preferable to use the median when considering analysis of variance and in particular lengths of stay.

In general, analysis is grouped by patient condition, although if a certain factor being analysed is common to many conditions, the results from all these conditions may be combined. For example, pre-operative length of stay is one day for many surgical conditions; this variable may be analysed for all surgery cases, thereby increasing the quantity of information collected. With a larger sample, variance trends can be more easily detected and reviewed.

Results of analysis of variation

The results of analysis will be different in different institutions, depending on the local priorities and questions asked of the analysis process. Yet there may be some common factors; for instance most analyses will include some or all of the following:

- Determination of the median length of stay
- Information on the frequency and causes of avoidable variation
- Details on the frequency and type of complications
- Clinical outcomes
- Analysis of patient satisfaction with the care provided
- Some indication of the cost implications of improved practices and services

Such analyses should also include enough information to enable the teams to develop solutions to the most important problems highlighted, or indications of where further information is needed. By analysing the problems which cause inefficiencies, local solutions can more easily be found. This results in the continuous improvement of services provided. Analysis of variance will help considerably to initiate change as it enables current practice to be accurately measured or quantified and then compared with what is done in the future. In this way improvements can be demonstrated factually or numerically.

Feedback and evaluation of results

Once the results of analysis have been obtained, all members of the multi-disciplinary team should be involved in assessing the results. Without a feedback process, analysis of variance is of little value. The way in which results are disseminated will vary, from written reports to presentations for teams. Locally produced credible and relevant information is more likely to lead to local improvements as it acts as a basis for changes in practice by the local teams themselves, making the local teams instrumental in implementing the changes.

Redefine Pathways

The quality of patient care delivered through the Pathway can continuously improve only if the Pathway itself is revised or redefined to incorporate the changes agreed by the local teams. In this way any changes proposed can be rapidly integrated into the process of care delivery for subsequent cases without delay. Such changes in practice can then be evaluated as further analysis is performed on these subsequent cases, thereby providing a continuous cycle of review and change.

Clinical audit and Pathways of Care

Clinical audit is by definition multi-disciplinary, involving review of the process and outcome of clinical practice. The first stage of the audit cycle defines the expectations or standards agreed by local professional teams in the planning stage (Fig. 3.4). The drafting of a Pathway for specific conditions equates with this part of the audit cycle (Fig. 3.5). The Pathway is then implemented into clinical practice and the analysis of variation from that Pathway shows the difference between what was expected to happen and what actually took place. This is similar to the part of the audit cycle that compares expectations or standard with the observed reality of practice. By determining the avoidable causes of variation from a Pathway and developing solutions, change can then be initiated. The Pathway is then redefined

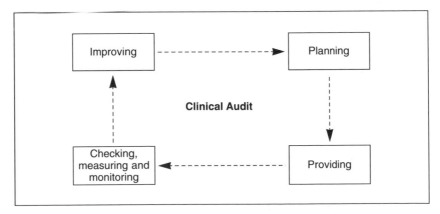

Fig. 3.4   The clinical audit cycle (NHS Training Directorate 1994).

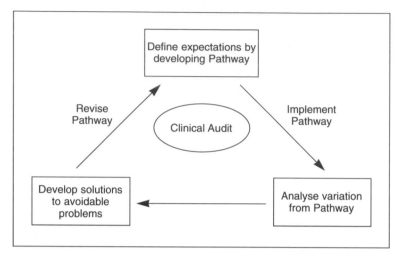

Fig. 3.5   A Pathway cycle.

in the light of the most recent experiences and evidence, equating with the completion of the traditional audit cycle.

Thus it is possible to implement the audit cycle as part of routine clinical care for the majority of patients, by integrating the audit process with the Pathway process.

Conclusion

Clinical audit and continuous quality improvement techniques are important aspects of health care which have been recently introduced in an effort to improve the quality of patient care. If Pathways of Care are used in conjunction with the analysis of variation they provide a powerful audit tool which constantly monitors the care provided. Clinical outcomes and the quality of care can be improved through the reduction in variation of clinical practice. These improvements are rapidly achieved by continuously revising the Pathway to reflect best local practice, based on evidence. Pathways facilitate the inclusion of clinical audit and quality improvement into routine clinical care.

Analysis of variation from the expected Pathway is an essential part of the use of Pathways of Care in clinical practice.

References

Coffey, R.J., Richards, J.S., Remmert, C.S., LeRoy, S.S., Schoville, R.R. & Baldwin, P.J. (1992) An introduction to critical paths. *Quality Management in Healthcare*, **1**, 45–54.

Hart, R. & Musfeldt, C. (1992) MD-directed critical pathways; it's time. *Hospitals*, **66**, 56.

James, B.C. (1993) Implementing practice guidelines through clinical quality improvement. *Hospital Management Review*, 3, 7.

Keillor, G. (1994) *The Book of Guys*. Faber & Faber, London.

Kendall, M.G., Stuart, A. & Ord, J.K. (1983) *The Advanced Theory of Statistics*, 4th ed., Griffin, London.

NHS Training Directorate (1994) *Getting Ahead with Clinical Audit; a Facilitator's Guide*. NHS Training Directorate, Leeds.

Rosenberg, W. & Donald, A. (1995) Evidence based medicine; an approach to clinical problem solving. *British Medical Journal*, **310**, 1122–6.

Thomson, R., Lavender, M. & Madhok, R. (1995) How to ensure that guidelines are effective. *British Medical Journal*, **311**, 237–42.

Turley, K., Tyndall, M., Roge, C., Cooper, M., Turley, K., Appclbaum, M. & Tarnoff, H. (1994) Critical pathway methodology; effectiveness in congenital heart surgery. *Annals of Thoracic Surgery*, **58**, 57–65.

Weilitz, P.B. & Potter, P.A. (1993) A managed care system; financial and clinical evaluation. *Journal of Nursing Administration*, **23**, 51-7.

Part 2

Pathways in the Acute Setting

Introduction

In January 1992 I was summoned to a meeting to discuss the implementation of Anticipated Recovery Paths (ARPs) in my speciality. I found myself with ward sisters, nurse managers and 'experts' from the Regional Health Authority. My initial understanding of what was being proposed was simply unnecessary additional bureaucracy. I could foresee little incentive to get involved, for it almost certainly meant more work for everyone and it was not at all clear to me what the benefit would be. Confronted with all of this, I adopted the usual tactic of a medical consultant under threat and challenged every notion that was put before me, be it a matter of the logistics, the people, or even the statistics. However, I did, albeit reluctantly, agree to participate in some initial meetings to establish whether or not we could put together an ARP.

Anticipated Recovery Path was the original term applied to the process, which is now known as an Integrated Care Pathway (ICP). A number of meetings were held during February and March of 1992; gradually the potential benefit of the process began to dawn. Initial piloting took place in March and April; and implementation followed in May. The process has been running over four years and is now accepted as the 'core directive' for the day to day management of every patient undergoing transurethral resection of the prostate (TURP). The benefits are now obvious to all staff involved, many of whom find that caring for a patient with a condition covered by an ICP is a less onerous task than otherwise. Within our speciality we have also created a further ICP for circumcision and are looking at other situations that may be covered by the process.

An Integrated Care Pathway works best with clinical situations which arise frequently – for it is only in those scenarios that full benefit is achieved – and in which there is a consensus of how to treat the patient in the first place. In the case of urology, the operation of TURP was an obvious choice. During the last five years our department has operated on nearly 700 patients at a total cost to the hospital of around a million pounds. Clearly, any improvement in efficiency in treating patients for bladder outflow obstruction with this operation, would be reflected in significant cost savings. More importantly, a structured approach in which better and more consistent care could be delivered, would permit a large number of patients to benefit. Above all else the patient must be the principal beneficiary of the process; however, if as a spin-off the hospital can undertake that process more efficiently and economically, then more patients can be offered treatment.

The operation

Transurethral resection of the prostate (TURP) is currently the standard operation for patients with a restriction of the outflow path from the bladder due to enlargement of the prostate gland (Table 4.1). They generally suffer from a slow stream, frequent and hesitant urination, a sense of urgency to pass water and dribbling at the end of the stream. Most patients present with these symptoms of 'prostatism' although some will develop urinary retention. The operation is undertaken either under epidural anaesthesia, in which case they are anaesthetised from the waist down and may remain awake throughout the operation, or general anaesthetic. An initial inspection of the urethra, prostate and bladder is made with a cystoscope (an inspecting telescope), and then a larger instrument (resectoscope) is passed. The operating part of this instrument is a U-shaped wire loop connected to a diathermy system, which permits either cautery or cutting. The enlarged prostate is reamed into numerous slices which fall back into the bladder and are then sucked out before the end of the operation. Cautery is used to control the bleeding but it is usually impossible to stop the bleeding totally.

Following the operation, a catheter with two channels is placed in the bladder; irrigation fluid flows down one limb of the catheter while the other drains the fluid out; this usually but not always prevents blood from clotting in the bladder or catheter leading to clot retention. Thus, there is no open

Table 4.1 Prostatectomy for the enlarged prostate.

- TransUrethral Resection of Prostate
- Undertaken for outflow obstruction of the bladder due to Benign Prostatic Hyperplasia (BPH)
- BPH is very common
  20% of all men > 60 years suffer some symptoms
- TURP gives better results than any other option
- Demand rising

wound anywhere and the irrigation is kept running as long as the urine is heavily blood stained. When it clears the irrigation is stopped and a spigot placed in that arm of the catheter; in our practice the catheter tube is removed on the evening of the first post-operative day. The patient then has to start passing water on his own, albeit across a raw wound. Once he has proved that he can pass water and without incontinence, then he can usually be permitted to leave hospital.

Developing the Pathway

The planning stage of developing the initial Pathway was protracted for no better reason than the difficulty of getting a large group of people together on a regular basis. As the ICP for TURP was one of the first to be implemented at Ashford Hospital NHS Trust, we were assisted in the drafting stage by Elizabeth Mullins and Denny Van Liew from North West Thames Regional Health Authority.

We put together a small working group to prepare the draft of the ICP. This group included myself, the ward sister and one of her senior staff nurses, a junior doctor (SHO), an anaesthetist (registrar), the urology secretary and a member of the medical records department. It is vital to ensure that everyone normally involved in the care of a patient undergoing the procedure in question is also involved at the ICP planning stage. It is easy to overlook admissions staff, secretaries and even anaesthetists. Everyone needs to understand that they must contribute and ensure the validity of the component of care for which they take responsibility. Only then can there be true multi-disciplinary ownership of the process.

It was at this stage that we realised an unforeseen benefit. The act of getting everyone together allowed us to discover exactly what the process of care for a TURP patient actually was. What I thought was happening to the patient was often far removed from reality. Furthermore, these early planning meetings allowed all members of staff to appreciate the role played by other disciplines and, in addition, everyone could appreciate each other's problems.

Three meetings were needed to produce the pilot document. The process is of an iterative nature; the draft cannot be achieved in a single meeting. Everyone needs to assimilate the important factors in the process of care and mull them over between meetings. Each member of the team trained his or her colleagues before the pilot ICP was run. It was then tested on the ward for a month and a number of relatively minor logistic problems were thrown up.

However, the most notable problem was that of the resistance of staff to change. As the whole process was quite new there was a tendency for nurses to keep their Kardex system going and for doctors to ignore the process altogether. It certainly took time for all members of staff to come to terms with the fact that, for the care of these patients, the operational document was a unitary sheet which stayed on the end of the patient's bed. Thus we learnt at an early stage that training and commitment are vital to success. The 1996 version of the ICP for TURP is illustrated in Fig. 4.1.

Implementing the Pathway

Once the difficulties had been ironed out during the pilot stage, implementation was relatively smooth and it certainly was not long before further benefit was realised. Shortly after admission, patients were introduced to the concept of the ICP (Table 4.2) and were told that all of their care had been planned out in advance; the staff nurse would spend some time going through the components of that process with the patient. This gave a clearly defined structure to the discussion between the patient and the nurse early on in the process of care; we were amazed at the level of interest shown by patients in the proposed care for them. Over the days that ensued, patients were frequently found looking at their ICP chart to find out what the plan was for them for the current day. When the patients' clinical course was uneventful, they would see a series of signatures and initials and found some comfort in the fact that they were conforming to the path of intended care for them.

Table 4.2   Features of an ICP.

- Document resides on end of bed
- Details all elements of care
- Replaces nurse's Kardex
- Patient's notes used for clinical narrative
- An initial to record care 'on plan'
- Variance recorded if not 'on plan'

I was initially concerned that patients who deviated from the plan would be more anxious, because they might feel that they had, in some way, failed. In fact, this does not seem to have happened and is, I suspect, a reflection on enhanced communication with patients that stems from the ICP process. Thus, if an event has to be deferred, delayed or changed, there is no option but to explain the reasons for that to the patient. He or she will then understand the reasons for that change and, in addition, usually feel that their treatment has been modified to meet the special circumstances of their case.

Results

Any departure from the Pathway has to be recorded as a variance, noting the nature of it, reason for it and who made the decision to 'permit' variance (see also Chapter 3 for the analysis of variances). The details of significant clinical change in the patient are still recorded as part of the contemporaneous narrative in the patient's clinical notes following the standard clerking notes and operation record.

Figure 4.2 shows an example of variance analysis for our initial ICP for prostatectomy. The single largest variance was of the irrigation to the bladder being removed earlier than the plan. This then led to the possibility of the patient being discharged early; however that possibility was only rarely realised. As a direct result of this observation the ICP was changed, so that the irrigation was removed a day earlier and the patient's discharge date was, likewise, moved a day earlier. Other features of note on this initial variance analysis revealed equal numbers of patients (6 each) suffering from prolonged low blood pressure and nausea. These events were noted soon after the anaesthetic. Such observations have permitted useful dialogue with our anaesthetic colleagues, to try and minimise cardiovascular instability following epidural anaesthesia and improve anti-emetic provision for those undergoing general anaesthesia.

A number of patients were scheduled for additional tests as an inpatient, which were unnecessary and delayed their discharge. A significant number of patients developed fever; some were treated by antibiotics (17 cases) and others not (10 cases). This observation led to a debate with our microbiologist about prophylaxis of urinary infection following TURP. Our antibiotic prophylaxis has now been changed and we routinely administer a single dose of gentamicin immediately prior to surgery.

The need for blood transfusion and the problem of clot retention (blood clots blocking the outflow of the bladder or catheter) noted on the initial analysis, highlight the risk of immediate and delayed bleeding after TURP. In this context the ICP process acts as a useful (and repetitive) reminder to the clinician that post-operative bleeding in these patients causes bother, discomfort and frustration for the nurse and patient and, in a few cases, danger. Since the ICP system has been in place I have certainly been a great deal more diligent in securing haemostasis during the operation.

It has also led to our consideration of the factors thought to enhance the risk of excessive bleeding, which we could influence and attempt to minimise. For example we usually try and rid patients in urinary retention

INTEGRATED CARE PATHWAY

EXPECTED LOS = 4 DAYS

PATIENT NAME:

TRANS URETHRAL RESECTION OF PROSTATE GLAND (TURP)

	ADMISSION DAY DATE — DAY 1	OPERATION DAY PRE-OP DATE:	POST-OP — DAY 2	1ST POD DATE: — DAY 3	2ND POD DATE:	DAY 4
CLINICAL ASSESSMENT	NURSING ASSESSMENT; ANAESTHETIST ASSESSMENT; DOCTORS CLERKING; CONSENT; URINALYSIS (if positive to nitrates - send MSU)	CHECK LIST COMPLETED, WITH BASELINE OBS AND WEIGHT.	IN RECOVERY ASSESS PATIENT'S FITNESS FOR RETURN TO WARD; RETURN TO WARD WITH WRITTEN NOTES; X-RAYS; DRUG CHART; FLUID CHART		CHECK URINE OUTPUT IS ADEQUATE AND THE BLADDER IS NOT DISTENDED	
TREATMENTS/ MEDICATION	PRE-MED PRESCRIBED; REVIEW CURRENT DRUG THERAPY & COMPLETE DRUG CHART	GIVE PRE-MED 1 HOUR PRE-OP AS PRESCRIBED; ANTIBIOTIC GIVEN ON INDUCTION	IN RECOVERY IVI & DRUG THERAPY POST-OP PRESCRIBED; ON WARD BP TPR RECORDED ON RETURN TO WARD; CONTINUOUS BLADDER IRRIGATION (ensure output = input); B.D. CATHETER CARE POST-OP WASH; 6° TPR & BP	DISCONTINUE BLADDER IRRIGATION (if minimal haematuria); 6° TEMP RECORDED; CATHETER REMOVED AT MIDNIGHT	GIVE TTAs	
IVIs			IVI AS PRESCRIBED	REMOVE VENFLON		
ACTIVITY/ SAFETY	NAME BAND (red if allergy); BED LABEL AS PER SURGEON	XRAYS/NOTES/DRUG CHART ETC AVAILABLE FOR THEATRE; BED REST AFTER PRE-MED	SPINAL EPIDURAL BED REST UNTIL SENSATION RETURNS; GA BED REST UNTIL SAFE TO MOBILIZE GENTLY	ENSURE PATIENT ABLE TO PERFORM ADLS INDEPENDENTLY		
DIET	NORMAL	NBM 4 HOURS PRE-OP	FLUID & DIET WHEN TOLERATED	FLUID INTAKE OF 2-3 LITRES	NORMAL	

		DISCHARGE
DISCHARGE PLAN	ASSESS FOR POTENTIAL DISCHARGE PROBLEMS	CHECK NOTES FOR ANY DISCHARGE INSTRUCTIONS	GIVE DISCHARGE LETTER & G.P FORM
	DOCTORS COMPLETE DISCHARGE / TTA FORM		
TEACHING / PSYCHO-SOCIAL SUPPORT	ORIENTATE TO WARD	TEACH PATIENT TC:	EXPLAIN TTAs
	INFORMATION GIVEN:	RECORD FLUIDS	REINFORCE TURP HEALTH EDUCATION
	a) TURP LEAFLET/BOOKLET	CATHETER CARE	
	b) DISCHARGE LEAFLET	REPORT ANY ABDO DISCOMFORT	PUT PATIENT DETAILS IN NURSE PRACTITIONER FOLLOW UP BOOK.
	EXPLAIN ICP		
	REASSURE		
RADIOLOGY/ OTHER	ECG		
	X-RAYS AS PROTOCOL		
LABORATORY	FBC	FBC (if needed)	
	U & Es		
	GROUP & SAVE		

Fig. 4.1 TURP ICP from Ashford Hospital NHS Trust.

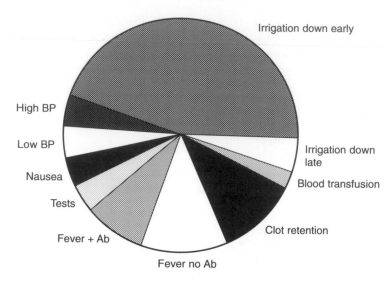

Fig. 4.2   Variances seen early in the study.

of catheters, even if only for a few days, before surgery; this allows inflammation from the catheter to settle and seems to lead to a 'less bloody' operation. We also now ask patients on regular aspirin therapy to stop taking it for seven to ten days prior to surgery; the proof that it enhances bleeding after surgery is hard to come by but there does seem to be strong anecdotal evidence, and personal experience, which suggests that it does have an effect on bleeding. The variance analysis has provided us with an indispensable tool with which we can better understand the process of care being delivered and also, by making change, improve it.

The attributes of analysing variances are noted in Table 4.3. It is a powerful tool because the data is specific, structured and objective. Thus it has a use, not only as a basis for refining the process of care, but also enables the process of audit and research. Records previously held in the notes, Kardex or other records were almost useless in this respect for, although analysis was possible, it was frustratingly tedious and time consuming because of a lack of any format.

An early feature of the variance recording process was to highlight the

Table 4.3   Attributes of analysing variances.

- Allows informed review of care delivery
- Provides source data that is specific, structured and objective
- Acts as a suitable basis for audit
- Permits comparison
- Enables research

degree of co-morbidity in patients undergoing TURP. Fig. 4.3 shows the percentage of patients suffering from problems with their heart and lungs, previous strokes, diabetes and arthritis. We had not previously realised how common these problems were among our TURP patients. In retrospect it is not all that surprising, as the average age of patients undergoing TURP in this hospital is 70 years. Appreciation of these problems helps in the care process. We now have clear guidelines for the care of diabetes in all patients undergoing surgery.

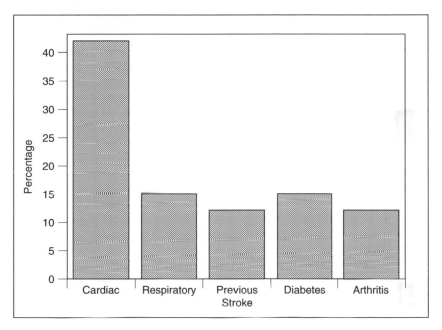

Fig. 4.3   Co-morbidity revealed by variance analysis.

Benefits

The spin–offs from the planning process were mainly as a result of every member of the team having a much better understanding of the overall process of care and the constraints under which other members of the team (especially the nurses) had to work. Several benefits resulted during the execution of the ICP process on the ward. Reduced paperwork was welcome. We were especially impressed by greater usefulness of the documentation because of its structured nature. There is also a useful educational component so that new staff, once they understand the ICP process, can see very clearly how patients with a given condition should be cared for in this hospital, as laid down by the multi-disciplinary team.

  If an ICP is being applied, then it is axiomatic that the plan of care is seen, by consensus view, to be the most appropriate. If that care can be consistently delivered, then the patients should benefit. However, proving that consistency in the application of care leads to benefit is extraordinarily difficult. However, there is one area in which a consistent approach can be shown to have measured benefit, and that is in the length of stay. Hitherto there were patients kept in hospital for no better reason than a lack of confidence on the part of junior doctors as to whether they should permit a patient's discharge. All too often they would insist that the patient stayed in for the 'consultant ward round'; there were also situations in which, over the period of a weekend, a patient was kept in because a team of doctors were reluctant to discharge the patient of another firm. Now, the nursing staff are empowered to arrange for these patients to leave hospital, given of course that they fulfil all the criteria, as stated on the Pathway, for safe discharge.

A new way of measuring length of stay

Traditionally stay lengths have been demonstrated by using bar charts. Fig. 4.4 illustrates the length of stay in cohorts of patients over three year periods using the traditional bar chart method. While it is clear that most patients used to stay from four to seven days, very little additional information can be gleaned from that chart.

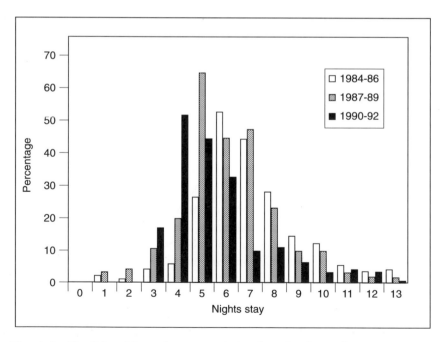

Fig. 4.4 Traditional bar chart to examine length of stay data.

In an endeavour to resolve that problem and make the analysis of length of stay easier, we evolved a technique by which the same data was expressed as a percentage number of patients still in hospital. Plotting this figure as a percentage of patients still in hospital against the number of nights in hospital, produces a curve, which we have termed the *patient bed dissociation curve*. Figure 4.5 shows a patient bed dissociation curve for the same data as in Figure 4.4. It is clear that between 1984 and 1992 the median length of stay had been reduced by about one day every three years (the point at which the curve crosses the 50% line is, by definition, the median length of stay; a much more appropriate figure to use in length of stay data than the mean). The points of inflection at the top and bottom of each curve indicate the period during which the majority of patients start leaving hospital and the point at which most have left. The tail at the end of each curve is a reflection of the number of people who have excessive lengths of stay. In these cases there is always some medical or social reason for the patient remaining in hospital. Thus, that part of the curve between the two points of inflection represents the discharge pattern of patients within a given population. The slope of the curve must then reflect the consistency with which people are sent home.

Figure 4.5 has, in addition, the curve for patients that I had cared for on a private basis. This was to make a comparison between what had been happening where decisions were taken by a team of doctors or by an

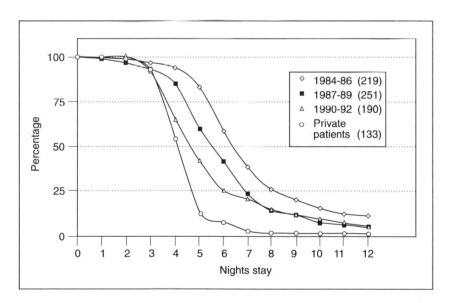

Fig. 4.5   Patient bed dissociation curves illustrating the same length of stay data as in Fig. 4.4 (NB: data from privately treated patients also shown).

individual doctor. The steeper slope of the curve for those private patients treated by a single clinician would suggest that there had been a more consistent approach than those dealt with by a team. Figure 4.6 illustrates our initial findings relating to 50 patients, before and after the introduction of ICPs, and this same pattern of improved consistency of discharge is clearly apparent. In addition, the median length of stay has been reduced by nearly a day. Figure 4.7 superimposes the pre and post ICP curves back on to the 1984–92 chart.

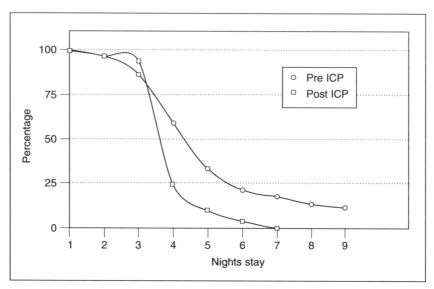

Fig. 4.6   Patient bed dissociation curve illustrating the effect of applying an ICP.

Conclusions

Despite initial scepticism I am now an enthusiastic devotee of the ICP process. Over the past four years I have learnt that there are many benefits to be gleaned but that there needs to be continuing enthusiasm for the process. By its nature an ICP promotes good communication between members of a team and encourages them all to work together in harmony.

An ICP without regard to the analysis of variances will stagnate; on the other hand a well managed ICP, in which lessons are learnt by careful scrutiny of the variance, will lead to the evolution of a well structured plan in which patients have the best possible care delivered in a consistent fashion.

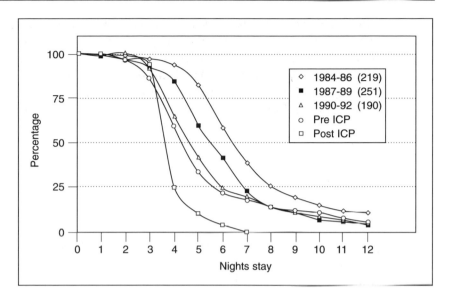

Fig. 4.7   Figs 4.5 and 4.6 imposed.

Acknowledgment

It is with pleasure that I acknowledge the tireless support of Sister Jan Paisch, senior ward manager. The success of the project owes a great deal to her vision and enthusiasm.

Chapter 5

Pathways in Cardiology

Louise Stead and Susan Huckle

Introduction

Integrated Care Pathways (ICPs) were originally introduced at St Mary's
NHS Trust within the Cardiac Sciences Directorate. This area was chosen
for several reasons; it was a major Directorate within the hospital, and the
successful implementation of ICPs in this Directorate would motivate other
areas to follow their example. The 'path' of a cardiac surgery patient has
clearly defined care parameters, such that it is relatively easy to predict the
trail a typical patient might follow. Staff within the Directorate were
motivated to be the first in the hospital to try out this new process of care co-
ordination. They viewed Pathways as a challenging and exciting innovation
and were eager to be seen to lead the way.

The Cardiac Sciences Directorate is also a high cost, high turnover
speciality. Pathways would be a useful tool for addressing potential problems in the care of patients in the area, and the analysis of variances from
the Pathways offered opportunities to identify areas where cost savings
could be made whilst ensuring that quality of care was maintained. Finally,
this Directorate had an enthusiastic clinical director, which was crucial to
motivate the medical staff throughout the developmental periods.

St Mary's was fortunate to be part of a pilot project initiated from North
West Thames Regional Health Authority, which commenced in October
1991. Since that time, the project has expanded throughout the whole trust,
although the Cardiac Sciences Directorate remains ahead of the field with
many more Pathways, both surgical and medical, now developed, including:

- Coronary artery bypass graft
- Myocardial infarction
- Percutaneous transluminal coronary angioplasty
- Insertion of pacemaker
- Radio frequency ablation
- Valve replacement surgery

- Stent insertion
- Angina

Developing the Pathways

Having chosen the area of Cardiac Sciences to launch ICPs, a period of extensive teaching was delivered. Teaching sessions were provided for doctors, nurses and all the professions allied to medicine (physiotherapists, dietitians, etc.). Each teaching session lasted one hour and they were held at different times over a three week period to ensure that all staff had the opportunity to attend. Training was delivered by the ICP co-ordinators based at St Mary's, together with the regional implementation team.

Right from the start, the whole multi-disciplinary team appeared to recognise the benefits that a process approach to care delivery could afford, and they welcomed the opportunity to improve the quality package the patients received. As in all situations of managing change there were some difficulties, although the positive approach to change by the team made these minimal and of little impact. There were two common concerns regarding the introduction of Pathways:

'ICPs will replace individualised care and dictate patient care'

Staff were reassured from the start that the content of the Pathway would be only what they, the clinical team, wanted; it would truly reflect what they were doing at that time in care delivery. Each variance recorded would make that Pathway individual for that particular patient. It was realised that each patient would react differently to a hospital experience, and through variance tracking the team would be able to record that uniqueness. Although the Pathway indicates the processes that are expected to occur, if a patient requires an alternative process or treatment, then that is acceptable as long as the reasons why an alternative or variation is required is stated on the Pathway. Professional autonomy is thus not removed; it is simply that the reasons for alternative actions are stated.

'ICPs will replace the Nursing Process and eliminate models of care'

The cardiothoracic unit followed the Orem Model of nursing. An assessment had been designed that incorporated this model approach, and this was made integral to the Pathway so that the Pathway complemented the use of the model. Patients are then assessed, their care pre-planned by the Pathway, and the evaluation of that care recorded within the variance tracking system. It is important to emphasise that the Pathway system can be adapted for the specific needs of the area where they are implemented. Pathways are a means to an end, not the end itself.

Coronary artery bypass grafts were chosen as the specific condition for the pilot, as they were the most common procedure performed within the unit. To maintain the impetus of the project it was important that results were gained quickly and fed back to the teams without delay, which can only be maintained with high throughput cases. The Pathway was written over four meetings, each lasting one to one and a half hours. Each meeting was facilitated by the ICP co-ordinator. Three consultants were involved in Pathway development, and they agreed to use the same Pathway between them, so came to a consensus agreement on the medical content of the ICP. Over time, the Pathway has evolved. Drug regimes have altered as the team has discussed care practices, and as staff have been appointed in new roles (for example, the cardiac rehabilitation nurse), this has had an impact on who delivers certain aspects of care outlined in the Pathway.

Implementing the Pathways

Following the success of the initial pilot over a six month period, the team decided to develop further ICPs in cardiology medicine. If a medical patient required a surgical referral or intervention, or vice versa, the whole cardiac sciences episode could then be managed on a Pathway. For example, a patient admitted with a myocardial infarction subsequently requiring coronary artery bypass grafting, would have his/her whole episode of hospitalisation managed on a Pathway.

Great enthusiasm for Pathways within the Cardiac Sciences Directorate has been due to the commitment of the nurse manager and clinical director. Such support and motivation has led to many more Pathways being developed.

Figure 5.1 shows the first draft of the myocardial infarction ICP, and Fig. 5.2 shows a more recent draft of the document. The reader can see how the Pathway has evolved over a three year period. One change has been with the signing for care given to the patient. Issues arose regarding accountability for care delivered and its recording on the Pathway document. Nurses wanted more than one space for each day to sign for care delivered; they wanted to have a box to sign for each shift. Other changes in the content of the Pathway have occurred as care practices have developed over time. If clinical practice changes, then the Pathway needs a re-write to accommodate these changes, so that the Pathway always reflects current practice.

Improvements in the quality of care also stimulate changes to the Pathway. For example, it was discovered that intravenous cannulae were being left in longer than was required, which held risks of infection and phlebitis for the patient. A prompt was put into the Pathway that cannula removal should be considered on a particular day in the patient's recovery. This drew the nurses' attention to the issue, and ensured that cannulae were removed earlier than before if it was appropriate for that patient.

As most patients on the unit underwent the same operation (coronary artery bypass graft), the team was quickly able to gain feedback from the analyses of variances, and the ICP team were able in turn to gain feedback from the local muliti-disciplinary team on the Pathway's reception. The ICPs soon became part of the unit's culture as the staff saw how their use can significantly contribute to improvements and upgrading of clinical practice.

The greatest problems encountered centred around two issues: signing for actions, and the recording of variances. In general, it is the medical profession that have the most difficulty in complying with completion of the Pathway document. The doctor's reason for this was that the Pathway was difficult to find amongst all the other paperwork at the bedside (drug chart, observation chart, fluid balance chart, etc.). Because of this all Pathways are now printed on yellow paper to ensure they are easily recognised and located by all members of the team. Nurses found it hard to pull themselves away from the tradition of writing patient records in freehand text, even if the patient's care had followed the expected plan. As already mentioned, this has been addressed with some Pathways including columns and boxes for each nursing shift to sign. Nursing staff appear to gain comfort from recording all their care meticulously, even if each entry is not actually required.

The issue of accurate documentation completion has been with us for a long time. During recent years we have found, in common with other hospitals, that 'documentation compliance is poor and becoming worse' (Addy-Keller & McElwaney 1993). The completion of the Pathway document is, for the most part, simply a signature, and this quick method of record keeping should help to improve the standard of documentation.

Each Pathway that has been written within the unit has led to fruitful discussion about, and examination of, practice of all members of the multi-disciplinary team as they work together towards the patient's recovery. Exchange of ideas and review of care continues as the Pathways are further developed and analysed. Within the Cardiac Sciences Directorate strong links have been formed with the pharmacy department. This department has embraced the opportunity for increased involvement in patient care and has highlighted how integral they are if the patient's care is to be truly holistic (Allen & Rainford 1994). This involvement has led to work being

Patient name..................

	Day admit CCU Date..........	Day 1 Date..........	Day 2 Date..........	Day 3 Date..........	Day 4 Date..........
CLINICAL ASSESSMENT	NURSING - ensure venflon in situ ADMISSIONS (W.C.) MEDICAL - clerking - refer to dietician if required PHARMACY review drugs in am	Nursing - bowel assessment - 4/24 obs Medical review Physio review Pharmacy review	Nursing - 4/24 obs Medical review Dietician review Pharmacy review	Nursing - 4/24 obs - bowel assessment Medical review Pharmacy review	Nursing - b.d. obs Medical review - TTAs written - Drs letter Pharmacy review
TREATMENTS	Fluid balance chart for 48 hours Written up - Diamorphine - Atropine - Anti-emetic - Analgesia MEDICATIONS SEE → Treatment sheet - ?SK ?TPA - ANTI ARRHYTHMICS - ? HEPARIN ? ASPIRIN	Consider oral drug regime	- Cease FBC if no failure - Daily WEIGH if failure - Consider oral regime Assess need for - HEPARIN and TRIDIL - Review interventions - PTCA - Angio →	Consider oral drug regime	Consider oral drug regime
IVIs	- IV in situ - Tridil Yes No		Assess need for IV	Assess need for IV	Assess need for IV
ACTIVITY/SAFETY	Rest in bed	Sit in chair if pain free Wheelchair to toilet Assist wash by bed	Assess for WHAM Gentle mobilisation Walk to toilet	WHAM to proceed if appropriate Mobilise Shower and bath with assistance	Fully mobilise
DIET	Full ward diet as tolerated				

DISCHARGE PLAN	Speak with relatives	Assess risk factors Assess social situation Start discharge plan	Assist need for sickness certificate Continue discharge plan	Continue disharge plan	TTAs/GP letter to be done
TEACHING/ PSYCHOSOCIAL SUPPORT	Assess spiritual needs	Give out S/K cards Educate and rehabilitation discussion with patient and family	Consider WHAM	Review WHAM ⟶	⟶
RADIOLOGY/OTHER	ECG on admission ECG with pain	ECG daily	ECG daily	ECG daily	
LABORATORY	U & E Creatinine Cardiac enzymes FBC Lipids Group and Save	U & E Creatinine Cardiac enzymes LFT Calcium PO4 FBC Clotting profile	Cardiac enzymes U & E Creatinine Clotting screen	Cardiac enzymes U & E Creatinine FBC LFT	

Fig. 5.1   Initial draft of MI Pathway at St Mary's Hospital NHS Trust.

Myocardial infarction

Patient name   Hospital no.

Care Category	Day 1 Date	Initials	Day 2 Date	Initials
Medical	Clerking Insert venflon Prescribe – Strepkinase Y/N TPA Y/N Aspirin Dose Heparin Tridil 50 mgs/Dextrose 500 mls Diamorphine Metoclopramide Other drugs as per protocol		Medial review including drugs Heparin	
Nursing	Observations 30 mins to 1 hrly Admission Assessment Cardiac monitoring Rhythm.............. Fluid balance for 48 hrs Assess spiritual needs Offer reassurance and explanation Pump available Y/N		Observations 4 hrly Weigh patient Bowel assessment Fluid balance 24 hrs Offer reassurance and explanation	
Pharmacy	Drug chart review		Drug chart review	
ECGs	On admission At end of thrombolysis On experiencing pain		Daily or if in further pain	
Activity/safety	Rest in bed		Bed to chair if pain free	
Physio	Referral		Physio review	
Discharge plan	Speak to relatives Inform patient of expected LOS Start discharge plan		Assess risk factors Assess social situation Continue discharge plan	
Laboratory	U+Es Creatinine Cardiac enzymes/lipids FBC		U+Es Creatinine Cardiac enzymes LFT Calcium FBC Heparin clotting profile	
Teaching/ psychosocial support	Reason for admission Explain what a heart attack is Cardiac monitor Why How long		Emotional reactions Feelings Fears Activity progression in hospital	
Ward administrator	Ensure old notes found Admit on PAS Print labels ? overseas status		Check ethnic monitoring Check GP is on PAS	
Named nurse AM	INITIALS ARE SATISFACTORY NEXT TO CARE GIVEN, BUT ONE FULL SIGNATURE IS REQUIRED PER SHIFT			
PM				
Night				

Fig. 5.2   1996 draft of MI Pathway at St Mary's Hospital NHS Trust.

done on the standardisation of prescribing guidelines for identified case types. The initial intent was not to change prescribing regimes; however some consultants have made significant changes in their prescribing activities because of the process.

Pharmacy intervention in the examination of issues highlighted by nursing staff (for example, bowel problems and nausea after surgery), has led to changes in practice with improvements in the anti-emetic and apperient therapies. Two specific areas have led to changes in practice which have brought the pharmacists much closer to the patient: counselling on the drugs that the patient takes home from hospital, and the advice given to asthma patients on inhaler techniques. The pharmacist has a much larger role in these situations on the ward setting than before, since the issues of inadequate counselling and advice giving were brought up at the team meetings when evaluating the Pathways.

In general, the whole team has found that the Pathways are welcome. The professions allied to medicine (physiotherapy, occupational therapy, speech therapy, etc.) have all found that the constraints under which they work, and the difficulties that they have, are for the first time being documented alongside the rest of the multi-disciplinary team.

Analysis of variances initially took place after the first 30 patients had been on a Pathway. As the volume of cases has risen, it has become more difficult to do analyses so regularly and for such small numbers. Analysis is now performed every three months. An epidemiological computer software package is used for the analyses. Complex questionnaires are easily manipulated and the recent addition of an optical reader that can automatically scan completed Pathway proformas has made the task even simpler and less labour intensive. The specific areas for analysis are determined through consultation with the multi-disciplinary team using the Pathway.

As more and more Pathways are developed, core issues are being introduced into the analysis of all Pathways so that these can be monitored throughout the Trust; for example, were particular assessments performed on time? The wards are receptive to this because any particular issue affecting several areas in the hospital can be picked up easily and a solution found. All information gained from analyses is fed back to the local teams using the Pathway.

Results

It is impossible to emphasise too highly the benefits of the 'increased level of meaningful communication between all disciplines' (Riches *et al.* 1994) that results from the work with Pathways. Other more tangible results include improvements in quality, changes in practice, and cost savings.

Improvements in quality

Although anecdotal, many patients have expressed confidence in the ability to question their care, with the Pathway as their guide. 'Patient empowerment' is a popular phrase in today's health care system, and the facilitation of patients to question their care is one way in which some of the power is being returned to the patient. Explaining the patient's care by going through the Pathway with them, and where appropriate with their partner or family, empowers the patient with more knowledge on what they can expect for treatment and provision of care. For example, patients will know that they are due for an X-ray on a particular day. This enables them to prepare for it, and also to question why they are having this test. If the X-ray does not then take place as planned, the staff must explain to the patient exactly why events have deviated from the Pathway. Thus the patient can be kept more informed regarding their care and treatment than with traditional documentation.

The Pathway is kept with the patient at their bedside, so that they can refer to it at any time. This means that they do not have to try and hold large amounts of information in their heads; they can refer to the Pathway at their leisure.

Patients' knowledge of their drugs, both on admission and on discharge, was shown as being limited. Since this was highlighted through the analysis of Pathways, work has been done to produce information sheets that cover a wide range of medications for each case type. This sheet is explained to the patient by the pharmacist, with the drugs not appropriate for that particular patient being deleted from the sheet. Thus each patient now receives an individualised information sheet regarding their drugs.

Practice changes

Discharge planning was noted as an area in need of attention. Since the introduction of ICPs, a 20% increase has occurred in the number of patients whose discharge planning really did begin on the day of admission. This improvement has had a knock-on effect of reducing the length of stay for patients undergoing a coronary artery bypass graft.

The Ellis patient bed dissociation curve (see Chapter 4) shows that for this group of patients, in the early days of 1993, the curve was shallow; then as the Pathways became more widely used, and the care more structured through Pathway use, the curve became steeper (Fig. 5.3). This indicates that more patients are being discharged on the expected day, such that the majority of cases undergoing a coronary artery bypass graft are all discharged within a span of two days. This can then aid the unit staff to manage

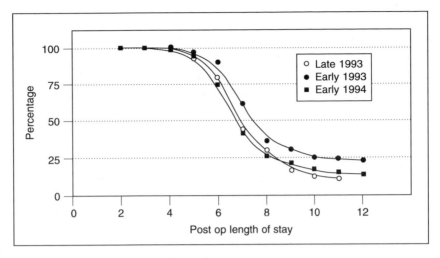

Fig. 5.3 Ellis patient bed dissociation curve applied to coronary artery bypass graft procedures during 1993–4, St Mary's NHS Trust.

the bed situation within the directorate, as they can be guided as to when a large percentage of their beds is likely to be free.

Use of ICPs has also highlighted the problems associated with the arrangements made for suture removal once the patient is discharged into the community setting. Inconveniences were caused both to patients and staff when there were difficulties in arranging for suture removal within local surgeries. As a result of the discussions around this problem, the surgeons decided to start using dissolvable sutures, and now there are no further difficulties for patients or staff.

Cost savings

The insertion of permanent pacemakers is performed on the Friday of each week. Once the pacemakers are inserted, they need to be checked before the patient is discharged, and with many of the regular staff not being on duty at weekends it often left patients in hospital over the weekend. This is costly in terms of cost per bed day wasted, particularly with the numbers of patients involved each year.

Since the Pathway for pacemaker insertion has been implemented, an agreement has been achieved between the radiographers and the medical/surgical teams. For standard pacemakers, the radiographer on call for the Saturday will check the pacemaker and if all the clinical criteria for a safe discharge are met, the patient is discharged home on the Saturday. This saves up to two days in hospital, saving money for the hospital and saving inconvenience for the patient. The precise cost savings for this small change in practice have not been calculated, although it has certainly eased the bed situation as the vacated bed may then be utilised for another patient.

The organisation of medication for patients to take home from hospital has also produced a cost saving. Many of the conditions treated within the Cardiac Sciences Directorate are in hospital for only a few days, with intensive periods of investigations or procedures being performed, all of which require the patient's drug chart to be with the patient. Drugs that the patient takes home need to be prescribed on a special form which is sent to the pharmacy dispensing department with the patient's drug chart at least 24 hours before the patient leaves the hospital. The drugs are then dispensed and returned to the ward. This has been extremely difficult to arrange as the patients are usually undergoing procedures or investigations the day before discharge, and hence their drug chart is required on the unit and cannot be sent down to the pharmacy department. As a result, the patients were often kept waiting on their day of discharge, creating inconvenience for them, until their drugs could be obtained from the pharmacy department. Some patients even had their discharge postponed over night.

Analysis of variances noted these occurrences taking place regularly, promoting discussion between the professionals. All agreed that the frequency with which this delay in obtaining drugs occurred was a significant yet avoidable cost to the hospital. Equally, delaying discharge of one patient will always delay the admission of the next. The team then set out lists of agreed and standardised prescriptions, and when these are used the pharmacy department will process the prescription without the drug chart. This has led to most patients being discharged with ease.

Conclusion

St Mary's NHS Trust have demonstrated their belief in and support for the use of Pathways, by making their implementation within the Trust an institution objective. The Trust acknowledges that through the Pathway process, staff are able to influence the future development of the care delivery process. Attitudes are changing, from nurse tutors to consultants to therapists. It seems that we are reaching the point where they believe that in order to adapt to new styles of organisation and management, they have to change the way they think. This, in a busy major London teaching hospital, is a substantial achievement.

Acknowledgements

We would like to acknowledge the support of Patricia McCann (Chief

Executive), Rodney Foale (Clinical Director of Cardiac Sciences), St Mary's Hospital NHS Trust Pharmacy Department and Nursing Directorate.

References

Addy-Keller, J. & McElwaney, K. (1993) A new documentation tool. *Nursing Management*, **24**, (11) 46–50.

Allen, L. & Rainford, E.D. (1994) Anticipated recovery pathways: a multi-disciplinary approach to patient care in hospital. *The Pharmaceutical Journal*, **253**, 30th July, 166–7.

Riches, T., Stead, L. & Espie, C. (1994) Introducing Anticipated Recovery Pathways; a teaching hospital experience. *International Journal of Health Care Quality Assurance*, 7(5) 21–4.

Chapter 6

Pathways in Orthopaedics

Kenneth Walker

Introduction

The society in which we live is constantly changing. Each decade brings with it changes which drastically affect the way in which we live and work. The last decade has seen what can only be described as a 'microchip revolution', creating a change in society of no less significance than the industrial revolution of the 1830s. Within medicine this has led to an increased ability to treat previously untreatable conditions, an increased life expectancy and with this, an ageing population. It is not surprising therefore that the cost of providing health care is rising exponentially.

The microchip technology has also given rise to increased expectations from patients using health care systems. There is now readily accessible information on the outcomes of their treatments, and sadly the pace of change has caught many physicians unawares. There is not only the need to audit work and to review outcomes; there is now also the need to contain cost if we are to continue providing the maximum amount of health care to all the population within a limited resource.

These challenges cannot be ignored. In order to meet such challenges there must be a collaborative effort from everyone involved in the delivery of health care to devise new and innovative methods of care provision and management. The Integrated Care Pathway (ICP) is one tool which sets out to achieve these goals.

The primary objective of the ICP is to enable the delivery of an agreed plan of care. There are two main goals that must be considered: the goal of the patient and the goal of the ICP. The patient's primary goal surely, is to be discharged from hospital in the shortest possible time, cured of the problem which brought them into hospital, or to be restored to health and free of pain in order that they may continue with their normal life. The goal of the ICP is to deliver a uniformly high standard of care to all patients, whilst at the same time keeping the cost of each patient's episode to a minimum consistent with the delivery of high quality care. In this way the wastage of valuable resources can be avoided, thereby increasing the number of patients who can be treated within the resources available.

Traditionally the consultant has been solely responsible for the patient's care, and quite rightly is likely to be somewhat indignant if it is suggested that he/she is not always delivering the highest possible standard of care. There is no suggestion that in using a case management tool like Pathways the consultant should lose clinical control of the patient. It is more a case of working with other professionals within the multi-disciplinary team to improve care.

That there is room for improvement in the way that patient care is managed is quite evident when an analytical view is taken of actual care delivered. Each consultant has his/her own concept of how they wish their patients to be managed, and senior nursing staff on the wards are familiar with this. How often does attention to detail in care fall short of the ideal? For example, an intravenous cannula may be left in a day longer than is really necessary simply because no one thought of suggesting it be removed. The patient is then at a higher risk of developing superficial phlebitis which is painful and distressing to them, and the treatment required incurs unnecessary expense. It is this kind of problem that can potentially be eradicated using Pathways of Care.

Orthopaedics is a surgical speciality ideally suited to case management techniques, particularly the ICP. The majority of orthopaedic surgeons in the UK hold a post usually designated as consultant in trauma and ortho-paedics. The proportion of each (trauma and orthopaedics) making up the post varies from one district to the next. The majority of the orthopaedic elective workload is related to 'cold' orthopaedic procedures, which are performed with a view to improving the quality of life of the patient concerned. The majority of elective inpatient orthopaedics consists of total hip replacements and revisions, total knee replacements and the removal of sequestrated lumbar disc lesions. Each of these procedures has clearly defined objectives, and is ideally suited to management by Pathways.

Developing the Pathways

Pathways do not happen. They have to be carefully designed and this requires a good deal of effort, not only with regard to the design of the document but also with regard to its implementation. Once the Pathway is implemented, there needs to be constant vigilance to ensure that it is being properly completed and used.

The orthopaedic unit initially developed three Pathways: total hip replacement, total knee replacement and fractured neck of femur.

The initial step towards introducing the first ICP (total hip replacement) in 1992 was to call a meeting of the multi-disciplinary team (MDT). This team was made up of all the personnel who in some form or another had a part to play in the care of the hip replacement patient. Members of the team included the orthopaedic consultants and their junior surgical team, the nurse manager from the orthopaedic ward, both a staff nurse and student nurse from the ward, the orthopaedic physiotherapist, social worker, occupational therapist, radiographer and pharmacist. This group formed the core of the multidisciplinary team, with many other members of the broader team being seconded when required (for example, staff from the transport office, or a community nurse).

The task for this team was to chart a typical hip replacement patient's progress, from the moment of admission to discharge from hospital. Right from the start the team had to keep in mind what the ICP was trying to do, and what it was offering the team:

- The ICP is a tool for managing patient care that will include the nursing, inter-disciplinary and medical process that must happen to the patient in a timely fashion in order to achieve the objectives of that patient's admission, within an appropriate length of stay.
- The ICP is a plan of care that lists the tasks and interventions that are required within a specific time frame, in order to achieve the expected outcome. Such a plan of care will also list the patient's problems and the actions or interventions needed to deal with these problems.
- The ICP is a teaching tool for patients and their families and for the orientation of new clinical staff.

The team also had to bear in mind the basic principles of an ICP:

- An ICP is patient-centred
- An ICP will identify the pattern of care required
- An ICP will reflect the pattern of care given
- An ICP will deal with the 'usual' patient
- Each ICP deals with one specific case-type
- An ICP will be used as a tool to co-ordinate, to track and to monitor
- An ICP will be used to monitor and improve the outcomes
- An ICP provides the average patient with a goal to achieve with regard to their progress and eventual discharge from hospital after surgery
- An ICP is used as a tool to enable proper discharge planning and bed management
- Each Pathway is ideally worked (within elective orthopaedic surgery) on the basis of a 24 hour module, of one day after the next
- An ICP is resource conscious

- An ICP is a valuable tool for audit and for research
- Developing an ICP must have collaboration between the various members of the MDT

The first meeting of the authoring team for this first Pathway lasted over five hours. At this meeting the various disciplines discussed care delivery for the hip replacement patient, and set out a day by day plan of expected care for the typical case within an agreed time frame. This plan was then typed up and distributed among the team members for further edits and comments, until a final draft was formulated ready to commence piloting. In the meantime ward staff were trained in the use of the document, as well as the concept behind the Pathway process.

When developing an ICP, one must consider how the Pathway can be integrated into the workings of a department, where there is more than one consultant team. The average sized orthopaedic department now consists of four to six surgeons, each of whom work substantially within their own team, sharing the beds on an orthopaedic unit/ward. Each consultant may have his/her own plan of care which may be different from their colleague's plan, even when the required objectives and outcomes of surgery are the same.

Developing a Pathway requires each of the consultant surgeons to sit down with other members of the team to discuss their individual management of the same type of patient. In doing this it is surprising how much agreement there really is. If there remain certain areas of disagreement between staff, then at any particular point within the ICP it could be stated that a certain action applies to Mr X's patients, whereas a different approach is required for Mr Y's patients; within this framework, the patient remains on the same Pathway for whichever consultant. This demonstrates the flexibility of the Pathway document for minor alternatives in practice.

Differences in management do occur when different consultants are nominally carrying out the same operation, but using different prostheses. At other times one consultant may insist on one particular procedure, and another insist on something different; neither has any evidence or reason to support their own opinion, yet they refuse to change their way of managing their patient, having followed this particular protocol for many years. For example, one consultant may insist that his/her total hip replacement cases stay in bed for seven days after the operation before commencing mobilisation, and the other may allow their patients to mobilise within two days and be discharged home much earlier. There is nothing wrong with alternative regimes of care management. Each consultant is free to manage their own patients in the way they think best. The problem will come when the outcomes of care are audited, and if there are no differences in outcome between those patients who are discharged much later than those who go home earlier, then the consultant with the higher cost per patient will have to find some way of substantiating his/her actions or be prepared to change practices.

At the present time vagaries of medical opinion are still tolerated, but with the development of the purchaser/provider market within health care provision, we are going to see the introduction of managed care organisations (MCOs) who will not pay a premium on any episode of care unless it can be shown that there is a significant improvement for the patient with regard to the final outcome. There can be no doubt that the consultants on each and every unit will need to work more as a team with other staff in their own units, if they are to be successful in competing for patients within a managed health care system.

The development of a Pathway does require a change of culture on behalf of the consultant, in that it rapidly becomes apparent that every member of the team can contribute, whether it be a student nurse or the ward manager, the house surgeon or the consultant, the physiotherapist or the occupational therapist. A typical example of this is when the house surgeon within our unit spotted that the product licence of a particular drug had changed, thus allowing a shorter period of usage with less cost to the hospital and a reduction in the pain and discomfort of further injections to the patient. This house surgeon brought the information to the attention of the rest of the team, and the Pathway was adapted accordingly.

It is this type of collaboration in the total care of the patient that ensures the quality of that care is constantly being improved, whilst at the same time the cost of that care is also under review. It must be noted, however, that cost may not only decrease; on occasions it may rise due to the adoption of a new treatment or a change in drug. When this occurs, it can now be justified with the ICP.

Implementing the Pathways

The Pathway document

The actual document used within our unit is laid out on computer and printed in 'landscape' format. Figure 6.1 shows a Pathway for a total knee replacement procedure. The chart is read with two A4 sheets one above the other. The first pages cover the pre-admission and pre-operative period, together with the operation day. The following pages cover the post-operative days to the point of discharge. Every intervention has to be signed by the attending member of staff.

When any criteria on the Pathway are not met, this is logged as a variance on the variance tracking sheet. The common variances encountered for this condition are listed on the variance tracking sheet and coded. This assists with automated analysis. Tracking of variances or 'variance analysis', as it is known in industry, has for many years been a vital aspect of any company's production, to ensure a high quality product. It is surprising that it is only in recent times that similar concepts have been applied in medicine, and yet the objectives have always been the same; to produce high quality outcomes.

Impact of analysis of variation

During the process of writing and implementing the ICPs, and then the feedback of information gleaned from the analysis of the variances, many issues were given the opportunity to be reviewed by the team, resulting in changes and improvements in practice. The daily observation and logging of the various criteria in the Pathway allows for early recognition of impending problems. With regard to joint replacement one of the most critical factors is the onset of any infection; this needs to be quickly brought under control should it occur.

One of the key issues with regard to infection is that everyone has their own opinion as to what constitutes an infection. This may be a simple reddening of the wound due to haematoma, or a full blown cellulitis. I am indebted to Professor Sean Hughes for his recommended definition of infection (Fig. 6.2). With the introduction of these simple criteria, the whole team has a much clearer view as to when a wound may be infected as everyone is using the same criteria. This definition of a wound infection is now written on the ICP, on the variance tracking sheet (Fig. 6.1).

Similarly, the early recognition of a chest infection or urinary tract infection is vital to prevent secondary wound infection when there is still a good deal of post-operative haematoma, and this may be identified early with appropriate assessments included within the ICP.

The analysis of variances will also pinpoint any delay to the patient's routine management caused by staff shortages or 'lack of availability'. If such problems occur frequently, the record of these instances on the variance tracking sheet provides documented evidence as to where the problem lies, enabling prompt management action to eradicate the problem. The same will apply to various departmental delays; for example, a patient may not be discharged on the expected day due to a lack of hospital transport at the weekend, or because the closure of the X-ray department on a Bank Holiday delayed the patient's progress with mobilisation. Information on such problems and delays enables management to take action appropriately.

The ICP document is not produced purely in an office; it is a customised

Patient Name :

(please delete) LEFT / RIGHT   Total Knee Replacement

	PRE-OP CLINIC Date :	sign	ADMISSION DAY Date :	sign	OPERATION DAY Date : Pre-Op	sign	Post-Op	sign
CLINICAL ASSESSMENTS	Doctors clerking		Make available : Notes		Commence fluid chart		Half hrly BP & P until fully awake	
	Operation fully explained by Doctor		X-rays		Operation site marked by Doctor		Pain assessment chart commenced	
	Consent signed		Blood results		Check X-match is ready			
	Weight ☐ Kg		Baseline TPR & BP recorded on TPR chart		Documentation prepared for theatre:		Nausea assessment	
			Seen by anaesthetist		Consent form		Theatre blood loss recorded on fluid chart	
	BP ☐ mmHg		Iodine sensitivity test done		notes			
					pre-op checklist		Wound drain is patent	
	Urinalysis : Glu / Ket / Pro / Blood		Result : ☐		drug chart			
					fluid chart		Review post-op intructions	
			Indemnity form signed		ICP			
			Waterlow score recorded on nursing assessment sheet		PCA equipment to go with patient to theatres :		Operation performed, and prosthesis applied :	
	Nursing assessment recorded		Review and complete nursing assessment		30ml BD syringe			
					PCA giving set		....	
			Urinalysis : Glu / Ket / Pro / Blood		PCA info sheet			
					All PCA equipment received in theatres		....	
					All documentation received in theatres		....	
TREATMENT			Shave knee if hirsute Y / N		Apply TED to non-operation leg		2 hrly PAC	
					Prepare Muller splint & send to theatre with patient		Mark drain at midnight & record on fluid chart	
MEDICATION & IVs	Prepare drug chart and send to Pharmacy via the D20 pharmacy bag, with a note of the admission date		Enoxaparin s/c 12 hours prior to surgery, given		Pre-med given 1/2 hr pre-op		PCA commenced	
			Enoxaparin prescribed daily for 5 days initially		Venflon inserted		Anti-emetic & analgesia prescribed	
							Cefuroxime IV given (x2)	
							3 units blood given	
							1 unit fluid given	

Fig. 6.1 Total knee replacement ICP at Ashford Hospital NHS Trust.

REFERRALS	Physiotherapist Social Worker if needed Y N	Inform physiotherapist of admission Occupational Therapist if needed Y N		
ACTIVITY		Physiotherapy assessment Practise breathing & leg exercises	Bath (assist if needed)	Bedrest
DIET	Encourage high fibre diet	High fibre Oral fluids encouraged	NBM 6 hrs pre-op	Sips of water when awake Progress onto light diet if tolerated
RADIOLOGY / OTHER	Chest X-ray Knee X-ray ECG			
LABORATORY	Full blood count ESR U & Es Group & screen 3 units			
TEACHING & PSYCHOSOCIAL SUPPORT	Give patient Knee leaflet Advise patient as to what to bring in to hospital	Orientate to ward Introduce named nurse Discuss knee leaflet, & check information is understood Discuss & explain PCA Explain ICP Discuss & explain operation		Complete prosthesis card
DISCHARGE PLAN		Inform patient & family of provisional/expected date of discharge (10 days post-op)		

Patient Name : ....

(please delete) RIGHT / LEFT Total Knee Replacement

	1st POD Date :	2nd POD Date :	3rd POD Date :	4th POD Date : ....
CLINICAL ASSESSMENTS	Waterflow score recorded Pain assessed Urine output recorded on fluid chart Wound assessed for infection	Pain assessed Fluid chart discontinued Wound assessed for infection PAC assessed	Pain assessed Wound assessed for infection PAC assessed	Pain assessed Wound assessed PAC assessed Bowel movements assessed & recorded on TPR chart
TREATMENT	4 hrly TPR & BP Wound drains: change if full mark at midnight, & record on fluid chart TED on non-operation leg Muller splint in situ	Remove bandage Remove wound drains Apply dry dressing & tubigrip Apply TEDs to BOTH legs Remove Muller splint QDS TPR	Dress drain sites Remove TEDs, & reapply after washing BD TPR	Expose drain sites & wound BD TPR
MEDICATION / IVs	PCA continues IV Cefuroxime (x1) Discontinue IV fluids	Discontinue PCA Prescribe oral analgesia *Codydramol, 2 tabs QDS/Dihydro-codeine 30 mg, up to 4 hrly/Ibuprofen 400 mg up to QDS/Naproxen 500 mg BD* Remove venflon	Oral analgesia given prm If opiates used, prescribe senna at night	Oral analgesia given prm
DIET	High fibre diet Encourage oral fluids	High fibre diet Encourage oral fluids	High fibre diet Encourage oral fluids	High fibre diet Encourage oral fluids
RADIOLOGY / OTHER	Knee X-ray			

ACTIVITY	Wash in bed (with assistance if needed) Breathing & leg exercises with physiotherapist	Wash in bed Leg exercises with Physiotherapist CPM 0 - 40 for 4-6 hrs Sit out in chair for short time Mobilise with physiotherapist and walking aid	Wash in chair Walk with Physiotherapist & aid CPM 0 - 50 for 4-6 hrs	Wash in chair Walk around ward with walking aid CPM 0 - 60 Active flexion exercises with Physiotherapist
LABORATORY		Check Hb		
TEACHING & PSYCHOSOCIAL SUPPORT	Discuss the operation & Knee leaflet with patient & family			
DISCHARGE PLAN	Consider for referral to Hospital at Home scheme If suitable for Hospital at Home transfer over to HaH-ICP	Review expected date of discharge with team Discuss expected discharge date with patient & family Expected date of discharge is:	Discuss transport home with family	Review need for Occupational Tharapy and refer if needed Y N Review need for social worker input and refer if needed Y N

Fig. 6.1 *continued*

Patient Name : ....

(please delete) RIGHT / LEFT Total Knee Replacement

	5th POD Date :........	6th POD Date :........	7th POD Date :........	8th POD Date :........
CLINICAL ASSESSMENTS	Waterlow score recorded Pain assessed Wound assessed	PAC assessed Pain assessed Wound assessed		
TREATMENT	BD TPR	BD TPR	BD TPR	BD TPR Remove TEDs if mobile
MEDICATION / IVs	Review Enoxaparin and discontinue if mobile Oral analgesia prn	Oral analgesia prn	Oral analgesia prn	Oral analgesia prn
DIET	High fibre	High fibre	High fibre	High fibre
ACTIVITY	Wash in bathroom Dress independently Active flexion exercises CPM 0 - 70	Walk with sticks & therapist Wash & dress independently Active flexion exercises CPM 0 - 80	Discontinue CPM Practice stairs with Physio-therapist	Walk with sticks unaided
TEACHING & PSYCHOSOCIAL SUPPORT	Review the Knee leaflet and check understanding		Discharge discussed with patient and family	
DISCHARGE PLANNING				TTAs written and sent to Pharm. OPD booked for 6 weeks Physio OPD booked Transportconfirmed : Hospital Family HV / DN referral made

Patient Name : ....

(please delete)   RIGHT / LEFT   Total Knee Replacement

	9th POD Date :	DISCHARGE DAY Date :	Date :	Date : ....
CLINICAL ASSESSMENTS	Wound assessment Doctor to assess patient's fitness for discharge tomorrow	Criteria for fitness for discharge no signs of infection apyrexial mobile with sticks pain well-controlled wound healing Criteria for discharge met		
TREATMENT	BD TPR			
DIET	High fibre	High fibre		
ACTIVITY	Practice stairs Fully mobile around ward	Independent on stairs		
TEACHING & PSYCHOSOCIAL SUPPORT		Explain TTAs Check understanding of instructions on discharge		
DISCHARGE PLAN	Check & complete discharge checklist	Give patient : TTAs OPD instructions re RTW in 2 days for suture removal DISCHARGE HOME		

Fig. 6.1 *continued*

VARIANCE TRACKING SHEET

Date	Time	Day on ICP	Variance and Reason for it	Code	Action taken	Signature

PATIENT CONDITION

1 Pyrexia
2 wound oozing/bleeding
3 wound infected (see definition opposite)
4 drain oozing
5 dislocation
6 nausea & vomiting
7 pain not controlled
8 DVT / PE
9 chest infection
10 poor mobility
11 constipation
12 UTI
13 poor urine output
14 mobilising faster than expected
15 frequency of micturition
16 catheter in situ
17 high BP
18 low Hb
19 confused
20 incontinent
21 Patient condition "other"

STAFF / PERSONS

22 doctor's decision
23 doctor availability
24 nurse's decision
25 nurse's availability
26 physiotherapist decision
27 physiotherapist availability
28 family decision
29 family availability
30 patient decision
31 patient availability
33 staff "other"

DEPARTMENT / SYSTEM

34 department closed
35 pharmacy delay
36 transport delay
37 laboratory delay
38 X-ray delay
39 community care availability
40 equipment availability
41 department/system "other"

Definition of Infection
pain at rest
raised temperature of > 36°
wound reddening > 2cm
wound discharge
raised WBC/ESR/plasma viscosity
NB: 3 or more criteria constitute an infection

Fig. 6.1 *continued*

pain at rest
raised temperature of $> 36°$
wound reddening > 2 cm
wound discharge
raised WBC/ESR/plasma viscosity
NB: three or more criteria constitute an infection

Fig. 6.2   Definition of wound infection (Professor Sean Hughes).

document produced for one particular orthopaedic unit. Construction of the ICP involved the formation of the MDT to produce a working document, which was then piloted for three months. At the end of this time the whole document was reviewed and changes made as necessary. Every three months there is a further departmental audit carried out with regard to the variance tracking, so that any problems may be highlighted and discussed. As a result of these meetings various items within the Pathway have been changed, and in this manner patient care is constantly being improved due to the regular review process.

As the team became more accustomed to the use of the ICP document, the writing of the later Pathways took less time. Training for new staff as they arrive at the orthopaedic unit has continued throughout the past few years; this is of particular importance for the junior doctors who rotate jobs every six months. All patients undergoing hip or knee replacement, or who are admitted with a fractured neck of femur, now have their care managed on a Pathway.

Pathway extension

The concept of managing care within the hospital environment is only one small part of the total episode of health care for the patient. It is the part of care one focuses on as it is clearly defined and is resource intensive. As such, the acute hospital episode is often the most frequently monitored part of patient care. Total Quality Management (TQM) of the patient, however, involves more than the hospital stay.

The initial period prior to admission to hospital is the first major area that needs to be evaluated. Frequently patients have been admitted to hospital the day before surgery, only to be sent home again with a previously undiagnosed or untreated medical condition. It is difficult to quantify the distress to a patient who is admitted to hospital for major surgery, only to be turned away at the last minute. Apart from the patient there are many factors which do not readily come to notice but involve other members of the family, such as taking time off work and making arrangements for young children. The cost to society of the social implications, although difficult to quantify, must be enormous. From the hospital's point of view it is probably too late to re-allocate the theatre time to another case at short notice, again giving rise to unnecessary waste of valuable resources. A little pre-operative planning could solve this problem, as demonstrated by the pre-clerking or pre-operative clinics that are now used in many hospitals.

The Pathway document has been extended to cover the pre-operative medical assessment in the pre-operative clinic. In this way we can ensure that full assessment of the appropriate and relevant factors is performed on all patients. At the same time the Pathway will guide the junior doctor to undertake the correct pathology tests and cross-match the correct amount of blood. X-rays and cardiac tracings may also be performed as directed by the Pathway document.

The pre-operative part of the Pathway, however, is not purely medical. One must never lose sight of the fact that the Pathway is a multi-disciplinary tool. The presence of the physiotherapist at the pre-operative assessment clinic is vitally important. They are able to instruct the patient on the exercises they will be required to undertake in the early post-operative period. With these clinics being performed a week or two before admission, the patient can be practising the exercise regimen during that time, and furthermore, relatives who come with them can also be instructed to ensure that the patient complies. It is this process of reinforcement which seems to work so well, and thus when a patient is returned to the ward from the operating theatre, they are immediately carrying out what is asked of them, without further instruction being required.

Also of vital importance is the presence of the nurse at the clinic. She can introduce the patient to the Pathway, taking them through step by step to ensure that the patient knows what will happen to them from the moment they come into hospital. The Pathway is carefully explained day by day up to the point at which the patient would normally be discharged. Thus discharge planning begins at the pre-operative clinic, with patients knowing at the earliest point when they are most likely to go home again. This enables the team to highlight problems which may arise on discharge, and thus deal with them early on in the admission.

The orthopaedic ICPs have also been extended into the community setting, (see Chapter 9) so that when a patient is discharged home from hospital early, with the support of a 'Hospital at Home' team, the same standard of care can be given to the patient irrespective of whether they are still in hospital or in their own home. It is not the purpose of this book to discuss the advantages of hospital care in the home environment, but the extension of the ICP in this manner is certainly providing extremely valuable information with regard to the problems and type of care required by the patient in the early post-operative period once they are back in their own homes.

Theatres

With the use of the ICP being accepted as part of the normal hospital routine, it was apparent that the one period of time when most interventions take place is when the patient is taken from the ward into the operating theatre. This is a minefield of inter-reactions between departments and individuals, and not infrequently delays and frustrations occur; despite many efforts it often seems impossible to ensure a smooth process for all.

Within our unit a pilot took place to tackle this problem for total hip replacement patients. The ICP was drafted to include the following areas:

- Transfer of the patient from ward to theatres
- Actions to be taken in the theatre transfer area
- Actions to be taken in the theatre prior to the patient arriving (checking of equipment, etc.)
- Actions to be taken in the anaesthetic room
- Actions when transferring the patient from the anaesthetic room to the theatre
- Actions during the operation
- Actions within the recovery unit
- Transfer of the patient from the recovery unit back to the ward

Figure 6.3 shows the theatre section of the Pathway that was piloted with the total hip replacement cases. This Pathway was part of the total Pathway document for hip replacements, being set in the middle of the operation day. This Pathway has not survived as it stimulated the theatre teams to develop a generic Pathway for all theatre cases, which has since been written and implemented and has therefore superseded the hip theatre Pathway. The simple listing, in a chronological manner, of all the activities and interventions that occur in theatre has created a patient record which in the past has been poorly documented, and is now easy and fast to complete.

Many surgeons may be disturbed at the prospect of having a protocol for the operation itself set out as part of an integrated Pathway of Care. The majority of operative procedures follow certain logical, sequential steps; each step has an objective and the only deviations in achieving each objective are the 'technical tips' which may facilitate that objective. Surely a much better way of teaching a surgical procedure would be to set out a

INTEGRATED CARE PATHWAY

Patient Name:

Total Hip Arthroplasty

Expected LOS = 10 Days

	PRE-OP CLINIC DATE:	DAY 1 DATE: ADMISSION	DAY 2 OPERATION DAY PRE-OP DATE:	THEATRE (PRIOR TO PATIENT'S ARRIVAL)	THEATRE Continued
MEDICAL & NURSING ASSESSMENT	DOCTORS CLERKING	NOTES AVAILABLE	COMMENCE FLUID CHART	CHECK EQUIPMENT IN THEATRE IS SAFE & ALL IS AVAILABLE	PRESCRIBE: FLUIDS / ANALGESIA / ANTIEMETIC
	OPERATION EXPLAINED	BLOOD RESULTS AVAILABLE		ANAESTHETIC EQUIPMENT CHECK	
	CONSENT OBTAINED	X-RAY AVAILABLE	SURGICAL SITE MARKED BY DOCTOR	THEATRE & SCRUB ROOM SET UP	COMMENCE PCA
	BLOOD PRESSURE	BASELINE TPR & BP			WRITE UP OP. NOTES
	WEIGHT	SEEN BY ANAESTHETIST	CHECK CONSENT FORM	SWABS/NEEDLES/BLADES COUNTED & RECORDED ON SWAB BOARD	2 UNITS BLOOD GIVEN
	URINALYSIS	SENSITIVITY TO IODINE TEST		INSTRUMENT CHECKLIST	HANDOVER TO RECOVERY NURSE
	MEASURE & RECORD TEDS ON FRONT SHEET	PATIENT NAMEBAND		**THEATRE TRANSFER AREA**	**RECOVERY**
		ALLERGY BAND IF NEC.		CALL WARD TO ADMINISTER PRE-MED	REMOVE AIRWAY ONCE PATIENT SAFELY MAINTAINING OWN AIRWAY
	NURSING ASSESSMENT	REPEAT URINALYSIS		CALL PORTER TO COLLECT PATIENT ON BED WITH MULLER SPLINT & PCA EQUIPMENT	RECORD TEMPERATURE
	PHYSIO ASSESSMENT	WATERLOW SCORE			5 MIN. OBSERVATIONS OF BP, P & SPO₂
TREATMENT		APPLY TED STOCKINGS		PATIENT ARRIVES ON BED WITH: MULLER SPLINT	WOUND & DRAIN CHECKED
		CLEAN GOWN & LINEN		PCA EQUIPMENT	PCA MONITORED USING PCA PROTOCOL
		TO THEATRE ON BED WITH MULLER SPLINT		TRANSFER TO TROLLEY	
REFERRALS	SOCIAL WORKER (IF NECESSARY)			WARD STAFF HANDOVER TO THEATRE STAFF, INCLUDE: - PRE-OP CHECKLIST - ALL PAPERWORK PRESENT & CORRECT - CONSENT	ASSESS FITNESS FOR RETURN TO WARD
MEDICATION	PREPARE DRUG CHARTS	CLEXANE 12 HOURS PRIOR TO SURGERY GIVEN	PRE-MED GIVEN 1 HOUR PRE-OP		INFORM WARD THAT PATIENT IS READY FOR COLLECTION:
IV'S				SIGNED: _____ WARD STAFF / SIGNED: _____ THEATRE STAFF	TIME:
PATIENT ACTIVITY	PRACTISE BREATHING AND LEG EXERCISES		BATH	**THEATRE**	CALL PORTER TO COLLECT PATIENT:
DIET	ENCOURAGE HIGH FIBRE DIET		NBM 6 HOURS PRE-OP	PATIENT TRANSFERRED TO OPERATION TABLE	TIME:

	PRE-OP CLINIC DATE:	DAY 1 ADMISSION DATE:	THEATRE Continued	RECOVERY Continued
DISCHARGE PLANNING	DISCUSS ANTICIPATED DISCHARGE DAY	DECIDE PROVISIONAL DISCHARGE DATE	CONNECT ANAESTHETIC MACHINE ECG & PULSE OXIMETER	HANDOVER TO WARD NURSE TO INCLUDE CHECKING ALL PAPERWORK PRESENT & CORRECT:
	DISCUSS ANY ANXIETIES REGARDING DISCHARGE.		POSITION CORRECTLY I.E. ON EDGE OF TABLE -PELVIS SQUARE -PELVIS SUPPORT ON -ARM OVER CHEST (JIG BOLTS ON OPPOSITE SIDE) - TILT AWAY FROM OP. SIDE BY 20° (NB - NO SANDBAG)	TIME:
TEACHING /	OPERATION EXPLAINED BY DOCTOR	WARD ORIENTATION	VITAL SIGNS CHECKED & STABLE	PORTER & NURSE ESCORT PATIENT TO WARD
PSYCHOSOCIAL	ADVICE ON ITEMS TO BRING INTO HOSPITAL	DISCUSS HIP LEAFLET	FLOWTRON BOOT APPLIED TO NON-OP LEG	ARRIVAL ON WARD
SUPPORT	EXPLAIN ICP	EXPLAIN ICP & CHECK UNDERSTANDING	CLEAN/PREPARE OPERATION SITE AS PER PROTOCOL	TIME
	H @ H SCHEME EXPLAINED	DISCUSS OPERATION WITH PATIENT AND ALLOW QUESTION TIME:	MAKE READY DIATHERMY, SUCTION DRILL & LIGHTS	
	PROVIDE HIP LEAFLET	EXPLAIN PCA	IF NEEDED, WASHOUT MACHINE	
			OPERATION AS PER PROTOCOL	
RADIOLOGY /	CHEST X-RAY		COUNT SWABS/NEEDLES/BLADES & INSTRUMENTS	
OTHER	PELVIC X-RAY		WEIGH SWABS	
	ECG		CLOSE WOUND WITH MAN-MADE ABSORBABLE STITCHES & 2 X REDIVAC DRAINS	
LABORATORY	FULL BLOOD COUNT		DRESS WOUND WITH MEPORE	
	E.S.R.		REMOVE DRAPES	
	U & E'S		REVERSE ANAESTHETIC	
	GROUP & SCREEN 3 UNITS BLOOD		DISCONNECT FROM MACHINES	
			TRANSFER TO BED & REMOVE CANVAS	
			APPLY MULLER SPLINT	

Fig. 6.3 Theatre section of a total hip arthroplasty Pathway. (Ashford Hospital NHS Trust.)

logical sequence of the steps involved. Surgical analysis of this kind could ensure a uniform standard of surgical technique, and when any intra-operative problems occur, the analysis of the Pathways would indicate the causes of those problems, such that preventive measures may be implemented at the right source.

The introduction of an Integrated Care Pathway is a major cultural change in the documentation and organisation of care delivery. The concept in any industrial organisation is far from new. In many complex organisations, a systems analyst will be charged with ensuring the company is competitive by looking at each part of the organisation and making sure that each part interacts smoothly and efficiently with the next to produce good quality results and outcomes at a reasonable cost. Analysis of variances ensures the continuance of a high quality product or outcome. It is surprising that the world's most complex business, that of delivering health care, where the expectation of its customers is to receive high quality care, has only just begun to embrace the methods which have been applied to consumer products for many years.

Results

Early analyses of the hip replacement Pathway showed that the physiotherapist was frequently not available when the patient required treatment. Closer analysis showed that this was occurring at the weekends and on Bank Holidays. The multi-disciplinary team discussed the analysis data and reviewed the possible options to enable the patients to receive therapy at the weekends. Joint replacement surgery was performed on a Monday, and the Pathway stated that the patient should be expected to transfer from a frame to sticks on the fifth post-operative day, which was the Saturday. The regular ward physiotherapist does not work at the weekend, there being only an emergency chest physiotherapy service, hence many patients had a variance recorded for the physiotherapist not being available.

Options considered included moving the theatre session to another day in the week; training the nurses to supervise patients' transfer to sticks; costing the delays in discharge and then employing an orthopaedic physiotherapist for the Saturday with the savings made from preventing delayed discharges; changing the system by which the physiotherapists work, and undertaking a shift system whereby physiotherapists work the Saturday in rotation. Each of the suggestions considered would cause the hospital great difficulty to implement, so the team then checked to see if the lack of a physiotherapist at the weekend was actually causing the patients to stay in hospital longer. It turned out that the patients were not being discharged any later, as they were effectively 'catching up' on their mobilisation during the following week.

The team then agreed that the physiotherapist, when visiting the patient on the Friday, would assess them and decide whether to transfer them to sticks a day early or to postpone the transfer until the Monday. The next analysis showed that the most common variance from the expected Pathway was 'physiotherapy decision'. This indicated that the physiotherapists were now making a clinical decision regarding the patient's mobility on the Friday as suggested, which accommodated the situation rather than causing great upheaval to reorganise theatre schedules or working patterns.

Length of stay has been reduced in all three orthopaedic conditions that have had a Pathway. The hip replacement Pathway was commenced in 1992 when the average length of stay was 16 days. This has been reduced to 10 days. The fractured neck of femur Pathway had been introduced for less than a year, when the average length of stay was reduced by 10 days. With the cost per bed day within the unit being approximately £200, for every 100 hip replacement cases a potential saving of £120 000 could be made, and for every 100 fractured neck of femur cases, a saving of £200 000 could be made. The earlier discharge of patients would also release beds for more patients to be admitted, thereby improving the utilisation of the beds within the unit.

An analysis of the total knee replacement ICP showed that one of the most common variances occurring was 'pain not controlled'. On closer inspection the team could see that this was occurring mostly on the second post-operative day. Total knee replacement patients make use of patient controlled analgesia (PCA), an intravenous system of delivering analgesia, under the control of the patient. On the second post-operative day the PCA was coming down, and the analysis was showing that the oral analgesia then prescribed was not being effective at controlling the patient's discomfort.

As a result, the team discussed recommended oral preparations with the pharmacist, and the newly recommended prescriptions were marked on the ICP document as suggestions for the junior doctors to prescribe. Once the next analysis was performed, the number of variances of 'pain not controlled' had dropped significantly, demonstrating that the control of pain was much improved as a result of the analysis feedback and the action taken by the team.

Benefits

Despite the logic of using Pathways in the manner described in this chapter, there remains a good deal of resistance to their introduction. The reasons for this include:

- Pathways require a major cultural change in working practice
- Pathways are perceived as time consuming, particularly in the developmental stages
- Pathways are perceived as simply more forms to be completed

For Pathways to be successfully implemented, there must be a perceived benefit to those involved. We have found benefits to the patient, staff and to the hospital.

The patient

A major benefit for the patient is that they become involved in their own care. The patient is always expected to 'help themselves', but how often has a patient actually been involved with their care? In the pre-operative clinic the senior member of nursing staff will introduce the patient to the ICP, which will form the basis of the management of their particular condition. The patient is taken through each day of their hospital stay and each intervention that will occur on each day. In this manner the patient is free to discuss any particular aspect of the Pathway with the nursing staff, and begins to get an insight into not only what will happen to them, but also the goals which they will normally be expected to achieve on a day to day basis.

How often has one seen a distraught patient concerned that something must have gone wrong, because in their own mind they had not progressed as quickly as they were thinking, when in reality the patient was quite up to expected progress. The only problem is that no one had told the patient how they would progress. Not only is the nurse able to take the patient through their hospital stay stage by stage, but they can also indicate at this early stage their expected date of discharge. If there are any problems which may arise on discharge, these can be dealt with even before the patient is admitted, if required.

When the patient leaves the pre-operative clinic, they are given a copy of the Pathway, so they and their relatives may familiarise themselves with the expected care they will receive on admission to hospital. Once admitted, the ICP is kept at the patient's bedside, so they can continue to read it. Patients without exception have welcomed this approach of sharing their care with them.

Staff/hospital

The ICP is now accepted as the legal record of patient care and replaces the ubiquitous nursing care plan, which although written by junior and often student nurses, has been accepted as a legal record. Thus, in real terms, the

ICP is not an additional burden of paperwork but replaces existing documentation with one which is valuable.

The fact that the ICP is a legal record has raised concern. The concern is that if there is a problem, or if the hospital are accused of a failure of care, then omissions or lack of action as a result of what may be documented could provide the basis for a claim of negligence. This does seem a somewhat spurious argument. The major problem in any accusation of negligence is the lack of documentation of what really took place. Any improvements to the documentation, which the multi-disciplinary Pathway tool offers, is surely of benefit. John Tingle expands further on the legal implications of Pathways and guidelines in Chapter 12.

As stated, the Pathway is the legal record of care and for nursing staff replaces the traditional care plan system with a much faster method of documentation. As the document develops to replace traditional medical and therapy notes, it will become a truly integrated record. The ICP thus facilitates a multi-disciplinary approach to care, and as such has the enormous benefit of every member of the health care team being involved and having an input, not only with regard to their own specific area of expertise, but where their interventions interact with those of other professionals, ensuring a smooth inter-reacting relationship between the various disciplines. Staff of all disciplines within our unit who have been involved in the development of the ICPs agree that they gain far more job satisfaction in this form of working relationship.

With the Pathway in place, the patient may receive a uniformly high standard of care at all times, no matter which members of staff are on duty. This can be important when locum or agency staff are on duty; with the Pathway to follow, they can deliver the same high quality care as the regular hospital staff would have delivered. The same applies to junior medical staff who are changing jobs every six months. It is common practice for the senior medical staff to instruct their juniors on the management of various patients and conditions, although the repetitive nature of such instruction frequently leads to various aspects of the care being forgotten or taken for granted. The regular departmental audits of the variances give every junior house surgeon at least one opportunity whilst they are on the firm, to sit down and discuss the Pathway and the variances recorded, allowing them to contribute to the upgrading of the Pathway. This is an extremely valuable introduction to modern case management.

To the medical staff the ICP can mean much more; it provides a valuable database of patients undergoing specific procedures, which allows the staff to carry out periodic audits and outcome studies, and even to write research papers without having to resort to traditional audit data collation techniques and reviewing of case notes.

The introduction of electronic scanning of variance data has enabled this task of analysis to be much faster and less labour-intensive, as the manual input of such data is time consuming and therefore expensive. Importing this data into a suitable statistical computer program facilitates the rapid analysis of this data.

Conclusion

The cost of health care provision is rising exponentially. The many factors for this have been well debated and it is not the purpose of this book to discuss these. However, the one factor which is undisputed is that unless costs can be contained, neither the country not the individual will be able to afford the continuing high level of care which in the past has been accepted as a right. In order that costs can be contained the various health agencies, both in the private and public sectors, have been looking towards managing care costs effectively whilst at the same time maintaining quality.

In the United States, Managed Care Organistions (MCOs) are commonplace, and in the UK we are now beginning to realise that the same methods of patient care are being applied here too. The Integrated Care Pathway is, in fact, one small facet within an MCO for the delivery of health care. This chapter has outlined the many advantages and benefits to the patient and the health care team of using an ICP. Indeed the introduction of the managed care concept has highlighted many areas where the level of patient care had fallen below that which one would normally wish to provide.

There is no doubt that district general hospitals, built on the Nightingale principal, are rapidly being relegated to the history books. Patient care will be bought, possibly from a hospital, with medical staff employed not as we know today, but on a contract basis for a particular job or session. The same medical staff may be in private practice and may be contracted to other hospitals too.

That changes in the delivery of health care and medical practice are taking place is without question. The direction in which these changes finally stabilise is unknown. There is, however, no doubt that medical staff who have the ultimate responsibility for providing care to each patient will, in the future, be required to substantiate that each patient is receiving the highest standard of care, provide an audit of the outcomes of their work, and maintain a low competitive cost per patient. The increasing use of Pathways is a valuable tool to enable the medical staff to take on this challenge, and working within these frameworks to provide a dynamic platform within which changes can be made and outcome constantly audited.

Chapter 7

Pathways in Paediatrics

Denise Kitchiner and Alison Harper

This chapter looks at paediatric Pathways from two different hospitals within the UK: the Royal Liverpool Children's NHS Trust and Ashford Hospital NHS Trust, Middlesex. Thus the chapter is divided into two sections, the first covering the experiences from Liverpool within their paediatric cardiology unit, and the second looking at the Ashford experiences within their general paediatric ward.

Paediatric Pathways at the Royal Liverpool Children's NHS Trust

Introduction

Integrated Care Pathways (ICPs) define the expected course of events in the care of a patient with a specific condition, within a set timescale. Any deviation from the Pathway is questioned, and avoidable variation prevented for future episodes of care, or corrected quickly and efficiently. Pathways use clinical guidelines that represent current best local practice. They can also incorporate evidence-based medicine and benchmarking (Shane 1995). Pathways facilitate the implementation of guidelines into clinical practice, as they form part of the record of care for each patient, and can be referred to throughout the patient's episode of care.

As the use of Pathways has become more widespread, they have been developed for use in paediatric practice. As in other clinical disciplines, Pathways are most easily implemented when there are established routines of care. The first Pathways to be developed are usually those for relatively straightforward conditions, where there is little variation between patients. In general, Pathways seem easier to develop in surgical specialities than in medical ones. This may be because the variation between patients tends to be less in surgical cases, particularly in those admitted for elective procedures. It is therefore no coincidence that in paediatrics Pathways have been developed more commonly for surgical conditions.

Pathways are usually unique to the institution in which they are developed, and reflect the best local practice. However, exchange of information between health professionals using similar Pathways can be extremely valuable to improve and extend their use.

Developing the Pathways

The methods of developing Pathways in paediatrics are the same as in other specialities, and the need to analyse the variances is similarly important. What is included in a Pathway will depend on the choices of each individual institution. However, within this speciality the Pathway should emphasise information that should be given to parents about what they can do for their child to encourage progress. There is little published in the literature on the use of Pathways in paediatrics (Crummette & Boatwright 1991; Weinstein 1991; Challinor 1992), therefore it is necessary to review situations where Pathways have been used successfully in practice, and to draw conclusions from these.

We have found Pathways of Care to work well in surgery for congenital heart disease. Pathways were introduced to the cardiac unit at the Royal Liverpool Children's NHS Trust in July 1994. Three conditions were chosen for the pilots: the elective surgical correction of atrial septal defect, ventricular septal defect and Fallot's tetralogy. The cardiac unit was the ideal setting for their development as teamwork and well-defined protocols were already in place.

The cardiac team consists of cardiologists, cardiac surgeons and anaesthetists, together with junior medical staff. Nursing staff on the ward and intensive care unit, physiological measurement technicians, radiographers, pharmacists, physiotherapists, dietitians and social workers are also part of the team. One member of the cardiac team reviewed the case notes of the last ten patients who underwent each of these chosen conditions. From the details of every aspect of care management, a Pathway was developed for each condition based on the median experiences of the patients whose notes were reviewed.

The provisional Pathways were circulated and team members asked for their comments and suggestions. A meeting was held and the draft Pathway documents discussed and amended according to these comments. From these drafts a final version of each Pathway was constructed, and the trial run was implemented. From the outset there was enthusiastic co-operation and support from all members of staff involved.

Implementing the Pathways

A full-time Pathway co-ordinator was appointed to supervise the use of the Pathways within the cardiac unit. The role covered:

- training of staff in the use of the Pathway document
- the daily review of patients on Pathways
- explanation of the Pathway to both patients and their families
- regular liaison with the doctor overseeing the system
- analysis of variation and feedback of data to the teams
- development and implementation of further Pathways

Reviewing the patients and their daily care enables a rapid response to avoidable variations from optimum care, preventing delays and reducing undue extensions in length of stay in the intensive care unit or on the ward. The co-ordinator also played a major part in the driving of the new Pathway system, to maintain motivation and enthusiasm from all disciplines within the unit. As paediatric cardiology is a high cost, high risk speciality, the use of a co-ordinator is justified, to minimise the risks and inappropriate costs of care.

Figure 7.1 shows one Pathway used within the unit for secumdum ASD repair, covering the pre-admission clinic to the day of discharge, with the variance analysis sheet where variances to the expected Pathway are documented for each day.

Results

The first 31 patients on the selected Pathways acted as pilot cases and were analysed in great detail to help with the fine tuning of a revised document in the further development of the Pathway. Variation from the anticipated Pathways, once they were fully implemented in that setting, were then analysed for 139 cases on the three ICPs for the surgical correction of atrial septal defect, ventricular septal defect and Fallot's tetralogy.

The Pathways contained a large amount of information and the team felt that it would be unproductive to analyse variation from every aspect of care. Therefore key issues were chosen for the initial analysis. These included the length of stay in hospital before operation, the length of stay in the intensive care unit, and the length of stay on the ward after operation until discharge.

Other aspects of care that were analysed included the duration of ventilation, the length of time before feeding was recommenced after the operation, and the amount and type of analgesia given on the two days post-operation. Any variance from the expected care was classified as 'avoidable', 'unavoidable' or a combination of both. Variations were classified as being

Please use this **Variation Analysis Sheet** to document any changes / variances from the pathway of care. Reasons must be given for variances as well as the action taken.

Variances may be positive (where a patient progresses more quickly than expected), or negative (where progress is slower than average).

DAY OF ADMISSION/PRE-ADMISSION CLINIC

Variance and Reason	Action Taken	Sign

PRE-OP DAY

Variance and Reason	Action Taken	Sign

NAME OF PATIENT ....

PRE-ADMISSION CLINIC DATE __ / __ / __
(or ward admission if missed pre-admission clinic)   DATE __ / __ / __   PRE-OP DAY   DATE __ / __ / __

INFORMATION TO FAMILY	__ Seen by nursing liaison sister __ Pathway explained __ Health Visitor/ School Nurse Referral __ Ensure accomodation needs have been addressed __ Visit ward	_____ admitted to ward at _____ (Time) __ Orientate family to ward __ Assess information given & family concerns __ Refer to social worker if necessary __ Explain procedures to child and family and establish family's role __ Discuss pathway with family __ Visit ITU
GIT		Note special diet:-
FLUIDS		Free fluids. Type of feed:-
WEIGHT & HEIGHT	Wt: Ht:	Wt: On calorie supplements Y / N Wt < 3 rd percentile or recent weight loss Y / N __ If Yes, HISS referral to dietician
TEMP / INFECTION PROPHYLAXIS		Apyrexial Monitor temperature, pulse and resps 4 hrly Report any abnormalities to surgeon Order CIVAS antibiotics:- (Teicoplanin + Netilmycin)
RESP		__ Seen by anaesthetist __ ± Premed written
CVS	Clerked by SHO Previous cancellation Y/N Reason: __ Pre-op meds written up Pre-op meds: _____	In hospital for 1 day pre-op Y / N __ Examined by doctor __ ECHO seen by surgeon __ Surgeon to speak to parents __ Pre-op meds prescribed:-
INVESTIGATIONS	__ FBC, Profile, Coagulation __ Hepatitis B screening __ Crossmatch blood __ ECG & X-ray __ Throat swab __ Rectal swab or stool specimen __ ± Sickle cell screen __ All tests complete Y / N __ Coagulation normal Y / N	__ Drs to check and document all results __ Abnormal results acted on Y / N Allergies:
	__ Pathway reviewed by medical staff Signed: __ Pathway completed by:- Signed:-	__ Pathway reviewed by medical staff Signed:- __ Pathway completed by nursing staff Signed:-

Insert a √ in the appropriate space once care has been carried out
Leave space blank if care is still to be carried out
Write N/A if care is not appropriate

Additional pre-op care plan used for other patient needs / problem   Y / N

Fig. 7.1   Pathway for secundum ASD repair at The Royal Liverpool Children's Hospital NHS Trust.

Please use this **Variation Analysis Sheet** to document any changes / variances from the pathway of care. Reasons must be given for variances as well as the action taken.

Variances may be positive (where a patient progresses more quickly than expected), or negative (where progress is slower than average).

DAY OF OPERATION

PRE-OPERATION

Variance and reason	Action taken	Signature

POST OPERATION

Variance and reason	Action taken	Signature

NAME OF PATIENT .... DAY OF OPERATION   Date __ /__/__   **ASD**

PRE-OPERATION

		SIGN
NPM	NPM for solids 6 hours pre-op NPM for formula milk 4 hours pre-op & for breast milk 3 hours pre-op. Time: _____ NPM for clear fluids 2 hours pre-op	
PRE-MED	Premed prescribed for 2 hours pre-op i.e. due at : _____ Given at: _____ Emla applied	
PRE-OP CHECK LIST	__ ID band present __ Jewellery, Nail polish, prosthesis removed __ Consent form , Drug Prescription chart __ Xray films, ECG, Lab reports __ Transferred to theatre with the above at: _____ __ Give parent the opportunity to accompany child to anaesthetic room __ Transfer to ICU via HISS	

POST-OPERATION

CVS	Returned to ITU at _____ Notes written by Dr on return to ITU Chest drainage < 3 ml/kg/hr over first 4 hours Y / N
DRUGS	Antibiotics only Y / N Other:-
TEMP	Core / peripheral temperature difference < 2°C within 2 hrs on ITU Y / N
RESP	__ Extubated within 2 hours on ITU Time: _____ Encourage coughing after extubation
GIT	__ Offer feed 4 hrs post-extubation or NG feed 4 hrs post-op if extubation not anticipated overnight and haemodynamically stable Time first feed:_____
FLUIDS	__ Fluids 1ml/kg/hr __ Change from FFP to PPF when coagulation normal Urine output > 2ml/kg/hr Y / N (_____ mls on return from theatre and _____ mls/kg/hr first 4 hrs)

LAB	__ Tests done within 30 min of arrival on ITU Y / N
	Tests as listed only
	__ Blood gases with PCV & electrolytes x 1
	__ FBC x 1, Profile x 1, Coagulation x 1
	
	__ X-ray x 1 (within 1 hr)
	__ Swabs: Throat and rectal x1
	__ Repeat blood gases with PCV & electrolytes - after 4 hours,
	                                      - pre-extubation
	                                      - post extubation

SKIN	__ Incision covered, wound not oozing
PAIN/ SEDATION	__ Diamorphine for pain control & sedation __ Paracetamol prn for pyrexia
ACTIVITY	__ Responding to stimuli within 4 hrs on ITU
INFORMATION TO FAMILY	__ Surgeon to speak to parents __ Reassure patient and assess family concerns __ Explain plan of care to parents
	__ Pathway reviewed by medical staff Pathway completed by nursing staff Signed:- Signed:-

Insert a √ in the appropriate space once care has been carried out
Leave space blank if care is still to be carried out
Write N/A if care is not appropriate

Fig. 7.1 *continued.*

Please use this **Variation Analysis Sheet** to document any changes / variances from the pathway of care. Reasons must be given for variances as well as the action taken.

Variances may be positive (where a patient progresses more quickly than expected), or negative (where progress is slower than average).

DAY 1

NAME OF PATIENT ....   DAY 1   DATE __ /__/__   **ASD**

CVS	__ Change to hourly recordings of observations (TPR & BP) within 12 hrs on ITU __ Discontinue rectal temp monitoring once haemodynamically stable __ Central venous and arterial lines out __ Chest drains out within 18 hrs on ITU Time: _____ __ Back to the ward within 24 hrs on ITU Time: _____ __ EGC monitor: continuous __ Change to 3 hourly observations (TPR & BP) on the ward __ Discontinue saturation monitor on return to the ward
DRUGS	__ Discontinue antibiotics after 3 doses
TEMP	__ 3 - 4 hourly temp recordings
RESP	--- Nursed in room air __ Normal respiratory rate __ Encourage coughing Assessed by physiotherapist Required treatment Y / N
GIT	Encourage diet
FLUIDS	__ Fluids 2 / 3 ml/Kg/hr as discussed with surgeon __ Urinary catheter out with groin lines Urine output > 1 ml/Kg/hr
LAB	__ Tests as listed only __ X ray x 1 __ FBC x 1 __ Profile x 1 __ Blood gases with PCV & electrolytes x 1
SKIN	__ Incision covered, wound not oozing
PAIN/ SEDATION (SEE PROTOCOL)	Consider stopping diamorphine within 24 hrs on ITU Y / N Time:_____ __ Paracetamol 4 hrly commenced prior to discontinuing diamorphine (____doses given) __ NSAID's prn if appropriate (____ doses given) __ Chloral hydrate prn
ACTIVITY	__ Encourage moving & turning after extubation Show parents how to lift
INFORMATION TO PARENTS	__ Dr to speak to parents __ Explain plan of care to parents
	__ Pathway reviewed by medical staff Pathway completed by nursing staff Signed:- Signed:-

Insert a √ in the appropriate space once care has been carried out
Leave space blank if care is still to be carried out
Write N/A if care is not appropriate

Fig. 7.1   *continued.*

Please use this **Variation Analysis Sheet** to document any changes / variances from the pathway of care.

Reasons must be given for variances as well as the action taken.

Variances may be positive (where a patient progresses more quickly than expected), or negative (where progress is slower than average).

DAY 2

Variance and reason	Action taken	Signature

DAY 3

Variance and reason	Action taken	Signature

NAME OF PATIENT ....   **ASD**

DAY 2 DATE __/__/__   DAY 3 DATE __/__/__

	DAY 2	DAY 3
CVS	__ Discontinue ECG & BP monitoring __ 4 hourly pulse & respiratory rate	__ 4 hourly pulse & respiratory rate
DRUGS	Pain & sedation drugs only Y / N Other:-	Pain & sedation drugs only Y / N Other:-
TEMP	__ 4 hourly Apyrexial Y / N	__ 4 hourly Apyrexial Y / N
RESP	__ Encourage coughing if chesty	__ Encourage coughing if chesty
GIT	__ Encourage solids	__ Encourage solids __ Bowels open post-operation Y / N __ Suppository if constipated
FLUIDS	__ Fluids 90 ml/Kg/day __ IV infusion discontinued	__ Free fluids
LAB	__ Request 12 lead ECG and ECHO for tomorrow	__ Tests as listed only __ ECG 12 lead __ FBC __ ±X Ray __ ECHO __ Check results and document in notes __ Repeat or treat abnormal results
SKIN	__ Incision covered, wound not oozing	__ Dressing removed prior to ECG Assess need to reapply dressing
PAIN / SEDATION (SEE PROTOCOL)	__ Paracetamol qds (____ doses given) __ NSAID's prn (____ doses given) __ Chloral hydrate prn (_____ doses given)	__ Paracetamol prn __ Discontinue NSAID's __ Discontinue Chloral hydrate
ACTIVITY	__ Out of bed for short periods Encourage to move and sit out	__ Out of bed __ Encourage to walk
INFORMATION TO PARENTS	__ Explain plan of care to parents __ Assess transport needs for discharge __ Prepare parents for potential discharge on day 5	__ Give discharge instructions:- activities - antibiotic prophylaxis
WEIGHT	Wt	Wt: __ To pre-admission Wt, or 2 days Wt gain
	__ Pathway reviewed by medical staff Signed: __ Pathway completed by nursing staff Signed:-	__ Pathway reviewed by medical staff Signed:- __ Pathway completed by nursing staff Signed:-

Insert a √ in the appropriate space once care has been carried out
Leave space blank if care is still to be carried out
Write N/A if care is not appropriate

Fig. 7.1   *continued.*

Please use this **Variation Analysis Sheet** to document any changes / variances from the pathway of care.

Reasons must be given for variances as well as the action taken.

Variances may be positive (where a patient progresses more quickly than expected), or negative (where progress is slower than average).

DAY 4

Variance and reason	Action taken	Signature

DAY 5

Variance and reason	Action taken	Signature

NAME OF PATIENT ....   **ASD**

DAY 4 DATE __/__/__   DAY 5 DATE __/__/__

DAY OF THE WEEK _____

CVS	__ Discharge	
DRUGS	Hb _____ gm% on Day _____ __ Iron supplements if HB < 11.0 gms%	
TEMP	__ Apyrexial	
RESP	__ Chest clear	
GIT	__ Normal diet	
FLUIDS	__ Free fluids	
LAB	__ Check all results and document in notes __ Repeat or treat abnormal results __ If pericardial effusion on ECHO > 4 mm, consult Registrar	
SKIN	__ Remove dressing if not already done __ Bath	
PAIN	__ Paracetamol prn	
ACTIVITY	__ Normal activity	

CARE PLAN	__ Assess parents understanding of - discharge instructions
	                                        - medicine doses and times
	__ Drain stitches to be taken out by GP on day 7
	__ Letter to GP
	__ HISS referral to Health visitor / School nurse
	
	   Appointment date __ / __ / __	

WEIGHT	Wt	

MEDICAL
STAFF
	__ Pathway reviewed by medical staff
	   Signed:-
	
	   Pathway completed by nursing staff
	   Signed:-	

Insert a √ in the appropriate space once care has been carried out
Leave blank if care is still to be carried out
Write N/A if care is not appropriate

SEEN IN CLINIC   DATE __/__/__   COMPLICATIONS Y / N

Fig. 7.1   *continued.*

NAME	POSITION	SAMPLE SIGNATURE

Fig. 7.1   *continued.*

caused by the patient and their family, the clinical staff, the system within the hospital or the community.

A newly established pre-admission clinic performed all the pre-operative investigations one week prior to admission, thereby enabling the patients to be admitted on the day before their operation. Length of stay in hospital prior to the operation was monitored through the Pathway, and showed that initially 28% of cases had a potentially avoidable reason for being in hospital more than one day before the operation. Length of pre-operative stay of more than one day was then reduced to 3% due to improved attendance at the pre-admission clinic by the patients. Although this improvement was not directly attributable to the use of a Pathway, the impact of improved practice could be easily measured through the analysis of variation from the Pathway.

Analysis also highlighted avoidable delays in discharge of patients, usually relating to a failure in completing the pre-discharge investigations. Systems were then put into place to request these investigations early enough before discharge such that they did not then cause more delays in the future. Junior doctors were also made more aware of the expected day of discharge after operation, and decisions to discharge were not then delayed if the patient met the criteria for safe discharge. The median length of stay has been reduced by one day for each of the conditions mapped on a Pathway. Avoidable delays in discharge from these new targets were then further reduced from 23% of patients being delayed to 10%. All of these corrections of avoidable delays contribute to reductions in the lengths of stay for these procedures, which has a significant impact on the costs within such a high cost setting of care.

Young children are often unable to clearly express when they are in pain, and information obtained from the Pathways indicated that post-operative analgesia was not always being given regularly. A comprehensive audit of post-operative analgesia resulted in guidelines for such medication administration, which were then also incorporated into the Pathway. This led to an improvement in the number of patients receiving regular post-operative analgesia during the first post-operative day, from 71% before the Pathway was implemented to 100% with the Pathway. Similar improvements were also shown, from 29% to 85% of patients receiving regular analgesia on the second post-operative day once the Pathway was implemented.

Benefits

Whether the child is coming into hospital for a minor procedure or cardiac surgery, admission to hospital can be a frightening and confusing time for him/her and the family. This anxiety may be reduced if the child feels safe and has some understanding of what is happening. The use of Pathways of Care helps to improve communication between the child, his/her parents and the staff. Parents are provided with more information in the details of care that the child is likely to receive. Such information from the Pathway gives the parent the knowledge that they need to explain confidently to the child what is likely to happen. It also makes it easier for the parents to ask questions on details of care that may be important to them or their child, better equipping the parents to answer the child's questions when they themselves have a clear understanding of the plan of care. This can be of immense benefit for the relief of anxiety and apprehension. We also found that parents were more satisfied with service of care when they and their child felt more calm, confident and comfortable with that care.

When children are due for admission for elective surgery, they and their parents come for a pre-operative visit. It is at this time that they are introduced to the Pathway; the planned treatment and care can be discussed with them all using the Pathway as a reference tool for later consideration and review by the family.

Pathways enable staff to monitor standards that are set locally based on the achievement of best local practice (Parker & Cleland 1994; Delamothe 1994). Having the standards written in the Pathway facilitates adherence to these standards by staff using the document, whilst enabling the team to monitor standard achievements when analysing the Pathways. This has been shown to improve clinical outcomes (Weingarten *et al.* 1993; Maclean 1993) by decreasing the variations in the care provided. Pathways also identify patients who fail to progress as expected for one reason or another, and this enables early intervention to correct inappropriate deviations from the expected (Schrieffer 1994).

Co-ordination of the care between the many different disciplines prevents duplication of effort in the completion of records and treatments provided. Junior doctors take a full history when the patient is first seen and many of these details are again referred to by the nurse who is looking after the patient, rather than repeating the same assessments and thereby duplicating effort.

Delays in investigation and treatment are minimised and their causes identified. Investigations such as X-rays and blood tests are necessary before discharge; if the expected day of discharge is known, the tests can be arranged for a suitable period before this discharge date. For some cases, with a discharge due at the weekend, the tests can be arranged so the results are available even at the weekend. In this way discharge is not unnecessarily delayed simply because results of tests are not available.

Discharge planning begins on admission within the accident and emergency department, or at the pre-operative assessment clinic. In this way potential problems on discharge can be identified and resolved early on in the patient's stay (Westaby 1994). This is of great benefit when admissions are extended due to inappropriate preparations for discharge, when the child is medically fit to return home. Hospitalisation is particularly stressful for children and their families. It is therefore essential that they do not spend any longer than is necessary in hospital. Parents often have additional pressures, in particular other children in their care. Unnecessary delays in discharge can occur when the investigations that are required prior to discharge are not done in time. A number of studies have shown that the implementation of Pathways or a similar form of managed care results in a reduction in length of stay (Shane 1995; Turley *et al.* 1994; Brockopp *et al.* 1992), and this has certainly been found with the cardiac patients in Liverpool.

Parental involvement in care is encouraged in today's healthcare delivery and Pathways can aid in this, as the parent can use the Pathway as a guide to what progress is expected and what they as the parent can do to help achieve that progress. Information may be given to the parents regarding expected length of stay and progress towards recovery and discharge through the ICP, as the variances are clearly recorded and explained to the family (Westaby 1994).

Pathways of Care have a large role to play in the use and monitoring of multi-disciplinary standards of care (Crummer & Carter 1993; Shane 1995; Challinor 1992). Pathways develop from evaluation of current practice, evidence-based medicine and benchmarking, thus providing additional educational value to clinical staff. The team approach to developing and using the Pathway encourages communication between the different disciplines, resulting in the clarification and co-ordination of the overall plan of care for the patient. The checklist of goals for each day, as we have in the Liverpool Pathways, is a very useful tool in a busy unit, particularly for guiding the care of new or locum staff. The analysis of variances provides for constant review of practices which in turn lead to improvements in clinical practice. Such changes in care are then clinically led, and the process of review stimulates debate on different practices and encourages the integration of new research into clinical practice.

Conclusion

Pathways of Care are dynamic documents that are defined on information based on recent clinical experience and evidence-based medicine. They provide particular benefits for families of children in hospital, together with benefits for the child themselves and for the professional staff caring for them. Pathways of Care provide a caring and cost effective approach to clinical practice.

Paediatric Pathways at Ashford Hospital NHS Trust

Introduction

The ward is a busy general paediatric unit of 24 beds, catering for patients from birth to the age of 16 years. A wide variety of specialities are attended to, including general surgery, orthopaedics, medicine, ophthalmology, haematology and oncology. The ward philosophy states that the child should be treated holistically, meaning that emphasis is placed on the psychological and spiritual needs of the child as much as on the physical needs.

Integrated Care Pathways (ICPs) were introduced into this environment in 1993, as it was ripe for success at that time. The unit had a high turnover of patients so that any new Pathways could be completed frequently and analysis could take place regularly without much delay between each feedback; this had a large part to play in keeping staff motivated. Such frequent analyses also facilitate large amounts of audit data. A paediatric unit can always find room for improvement in the education of children and their families regarding the care they receive, and the team felt strongly that ICPs could help significantly in this.

Developing the Pathway

ICPs were first introduced to the ward in December 1993. A 'link person' from within the staff on the ward was chosen to act as local Pathway leader, and to liaise with the hospital's own Pathway facilitator. A middle grade staff nurse was selected; a more senior grade was thought to be too pressured with managerial responsibilities to be able to devote enough time in the development of the project. Also, the local team were concerned that information on the Pathway concept should be cascaded up and down the hierarchy, rather than just down from a senior member of staff. This strategy served the unit well in promoting local team ownership of the Pathways produced and their use within the unit.

The first Pathway that was chosen to be piloted was for paediatric circumcision. This procedure was chosen because these cases were regularly accommodated on the ward, producing high case numbers, and the surgeons of this procedure had been involved in other adult Pathways elsewhere in the hospital, so were accustomed to the process. Also, circumcision is a relatively simple operative procedure with a fairly straightforward recovery process in the post-operative period, and therefore fairly easy to map out.

Development of this first Pathway was easier than anticipated, probably due to the fact that a simple procedure had been chosen. Multi-disciplinary team meetings of all those staff involved in the care of the circumcision patient were difficult to organise, as it was uncommon for all staff to be available at the same times. To get around this the local link person spoke with each member of the team, and then came up with a first draft of the circumcision Pathway from the requirements identified. This was then distributed to everyone asking them for their comments and edits. The draft Pathway was also displayed on an ICP noticeboard that was set up within the ward, so that all staff in the unit, whether on the authoring team or not, could make their comments about the document and its wording and content (Fig. 7.2).

After two months the Pathway was ready to be piloted, so the link person set about training all the staff on how to use the document. Most training took place at staff handover sessions or when staff working in shift patterns had overlaps between shifts, and hence were able to be released for half an hour.

Initially some members of staff were very sceptical about the use of Pathways, suggesting that it was just another piece of paper to be completed. Once they were involved in the process of developing and using the document, however, they were soon convinced that it could replace much of the traditional documentation and thereby reduce the amount of paperwork, particularly for the nursing staff. It was during the training sessions that the motivation of staff increased and their suspicions reduced.

Implementating the Pathway

After a short pilot run of ten cases, to check the content and ambiguity of the wording of the Pathway document, the circumcision ICP was fully implemented, and then used for all admissions of this case-type. Every 30–40 cases the Pathways were reviewed and the variances analysed. This information was then fed back to the local team, either in team meetings or by displaying the results of analysis on the ICP noticeboard.

Each time the Pathway was reviewed and the results fed back to the team, the Pathway document was also reviewed. In the early stages the ICP was edited slightly following each analysis, but as the Pathway became more firmly established as a process of organising care delivery, the content did not always need to be edited, unless new research was brought to the team's attention from the literature and required the ICP to be updated. In this way the team has been able to ensure that the Pathway has been based on current evidence-based practice.

The Pathway process highlighted problems with the discharge of patients, with needless delays due to doctors not always being available to assess the children for going home, even if they had an uncomplicated post-operative recovery. The nurses discussed this with the surgical teams and as a result a set of discharge criteria were established, so that the paediatric nurses could take the decision to discharge patients themselves on the expected discharge day, if the patients met the stated criteria. There was also a related issue to do with different surgeons having varying views of what those discharge criteria should be, particularly regarding the inclusion of whether or not the child should pass urine prior to discharge. The surgeons and the nurses again had discussions about this issue, and came to a consensus agreement on what those discharge criteria should be regarding passing urine.

Such edits and changes to the content of the Pathway document are to be expected when the Pathway is young, and relatively untested. As the Pathway is used over a longer period of time the care becomes firmly established with local best practice, based on research evidence, and as such is questioned less frequently.

Results

The first set of analysis of the paediatric circumcision ICP was performed in July 1994. The local link person performed this analysis. Information was gained on the following issues:

INTEGRATED CARE PATHWAY

Patient Name:

PAEDIATRIC CIRCUMCISION

Length of Stay: 1 Day

	PRE-OP CHECK DAY DATE:	OPERATION DAY DATE:	
		PRE - OP	POST - OP
CLINICAL ASSESSMENT	DCD COMPLETED BY: NURSES: ANAESTHETIST: SURGICAL HO:		*IN RECOVERY:* AIRWAY CLEAR AND SELF MAINTAINED WOUND SITE CLEAN WITH NO BLEEDING CHECK CHILD READY TO RETURN TO WARD: RECOVERY NURSE: WARD NURSE: *ON WARD* 1/2 HOURLY P & R FOR 2 HRS DISCONTINUE P & R WHEN 'NORMAL' FOR AGE WOUND ASSESSMENT 1/2 HOURLY FOR 2 HRS FINAL WOUND ASSESSMENT IMMEDIATELY PRIOR TO DISCHARGE PAIN ASSESSMENT 1/2 HOURLY FOR 2 HRS
TREATMENT / MEDICATION	PRE-MED PRESCRIBED YES / NO EMLA CREAM PRESCRIBED: YES / NO	IF PRESCRIBED, EMLA CREAM APPLIED 1-2 HOURS PRE - OP, WITH EXPLANATION TO THE CHILD & PARENT(S)	*IN RECOVERY:* PERIOPERATIVE ANALGESIA GIVEN POST OPERATIVE ANALGESIA PRESCRIBED: POST OPERATIVE ANALGESIA GIVEN

	Column 1	Column 2	Column 3
SPECIFIC CARE	PREPARE NAME BAND (RED IF ALLERGY)	APPLY NAME BAND	NURSING STAFF COLLECT CHILD WITH PARENT(S)
ACTIVITY / SAFETY		D.C.D. PRE-OP CHECK LIST / ESCORT CHILD & PARENT(S) TO THEATRE WITH NOTES AND D.C.D.	FITNESS FOR DISCHARGE ASSESSED BY NURSE:
DIET	ADVISE PARENT(S) TO FAST CHILD AT LEAST 6 HOURS PRE-OP BUT ENCOURAGE FLUIDS IMMEDIATELY PRIOR TO THAT.	N B M	FLUIDS WHEN FULLY AWAKE AND DIET AS TOLERATED.
TEACHING PSYCHOSOCIAL SUPPORT FOR CHILD & FAMILY	WELCOME & ORIENTATE WHOLE FAMILY TO WARD & PARENT(S) UNIT / GIVE WARD INFORMATION LEAFLET / INFORMATION OF NAMED NURSE IN RECOVERY GIVEN / INFORM PARENT(S) CHILD TO ARRIVE AT 8 AM ON OPERATION DAY / ATTENDED SATURDAY CLUB — YES / NO / EXPLAIN ICP	WELCOME & INTRODUCE YOURSELF TO CHILD & FAMILY / EXPLAIN WHAT IS TO HAPPEN & CHECK UNDERSTANDING / RELAXED IN THEATRE — YES / NO	REASSURE CHILD/PARENT(S) / ENSURE PARENT(S) HAVE INFORMATION LEAFLETS & CHECK UNDERSTANDING / ADVISE PARENT(S) OF PARACETAMOL USE / EXPLAIN TO PARENT(S) THAT STITCHES TAKE 6 WEEKS TO DISSOLVE FROM SCROTUM ?DISSOLVABLE SUTURES TO INCISION
DISCHARGE PLAN	INFORM PARENT(S) OF EXPECTED DISCHARGE TIME AND DATE.		BRAVERY CERTIFICATE / GIVE WARD TELEPHONE NO. TO PARENT(S) FOR CONTACT / NURSE COMPLETED D.C.D. DISCHARGE / **DISCHARGE**

Fig. 7.2 *Paediatric circumcision ICP (Ashford Hospital NHS Trust).*

VARIANCE ANALYSIS SHEET

PAEDIATRIC CIRCUMCISION

PATIENT NAME: _____

DATE	TIME	VARIANCE AND REASON FOR IT	VARIANCE CODE	+/-	ACTION TAKEN	SIGNATURE

VARIANCE CODES

PATIENT CONDITION / FAMILY

1 WOUND BLEEDING
2 NAUSEA & VOMITING
3 PARENTAL ANXIETY
4 PATIENT UNCO-OPERATIVE
5 PARENT(S) UNCO-OPERATIVE
6 OTHER

PHYSICIAN/NURSE/PARAMEDICAL

7 PHYSICIANS DECISION
8 PHYSICIANS RESPONSE TIME
9 NURSES DECISION
10 NURSES RESPONSE TIME
11 PARAMEDICAL DECISION
12 PARAMEDICAL RESPONSE TIME
13 ANAESTHETIST DECISION
14 ANAESTHETIST RESPONSE TIME

SYSTEM

15 BED/APPT TIME AVAILABILITY
16 INFORMATION/DATA AVAILABILITY
17 SUPPLIES/EQUIPMENT AVAILABILITY
18 DEPARTMENT OVERBOOKED
19 DEPARTMENT CLOSED
20 SYSTEM OTHER

COMMUNITY

21 EXTENDED CARE AVAILABILITY
22 COMMUNITY SERVICES AVAILABILITY
23 AMBULANCE DELAY
24 COMMUNITY OTHER

Fig. 7.2 continued.

- Consultant distribution
- Age of patients
- Use of pre-medication
- Use of local anaesthetic cream
- Variances from the anticipated Pathway
- Errors in completion of the document

Consultant distribution (Fig. 7.3) showed the team how many circumcisions were being performed by each of the surgeons, and enabled them to collate variances from the Pathway with each surgical team. This facilitates the review of care as each team delivers it, so that if particular variances are commonly occurring for one surgical team, that particular team can be asked why they do not follow the guideline of care within the Pathway, and can review their reasons for deviation. The reasons may be perfectly valid and relevant for the procedure concerned, and as such, if there are valid concerns over certain aspects of care on the Pathway, then their concerns should be discussed more widely with the whole multi-disciplinary team.

The age of the children was also reviewed (Fig. 7.4), so that the team could ascertain what was the more common age grouping of children coming in for this operation. The ward had already set up a Saturday Club where they were inviting children to visit the ward before their elective

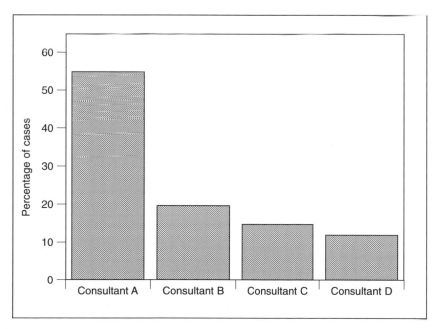

Fig. 7.3   Consultant distribution for children undergoing circumcision.

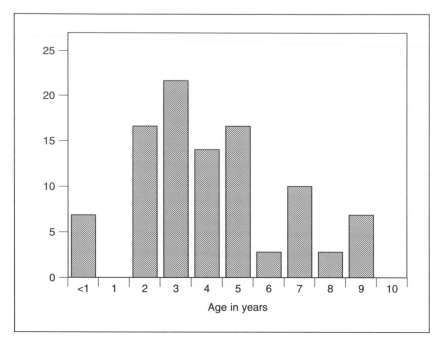

Fig. 7.4 Age distribution for children undergoing circumcision.

surgery. At this club the children were being taught what they could expect when they were due to be admitted. The level of this education needed to be pitched at the correct age group; the information gained from the review of the more common age groupings was useful to help the nursing staff pitch their education at the Saturday Club at the correct level for their patients.

For a long time now children have been having pre-operative medication prior to going down to theatres for their surgery. Such medication is meant to help reduce anxiety for the child, with a mild sedative being the most commonly used medication in this situation. The expected process with the child on the day of operation would ideally be for the parent(s) to be with their child, keeping them calm and comfortable. The child should then co-operate in taking the pre-operative medication without complaint, and then settle down and relax until they arrive in the anaesthetic room and are anaesthetised.

Realistically this rarely occurred! The children found the syrup tasted 'horrible', and it was difficult to get them to take it. Many children spat the syrup out so that the exact amount of medication delivered was hard to ascertain. Equally, the whole episode of giving this medicine was upsetting to the child and was not conducive to them being free of anxiety and relaxed. Preparation for surgery thus became a difficult experience for the child, their family and the staff. The nursing staff recognised a need for change, and a literature review was performed on the use of pre-operative medications for children.

Analysis of the circumcision ICP showed that roughly half of the children (47%) were prescribed a pre-operative medication by the anaesthetists, and the other half were not (Fig. 7.5). The literature provided no conclusive evidence that it was better or worse for the child to have a pre-operative medication, simply saying that 'the international literature on children hospitalised for surgery suggests that all children need some kind of psychological preparation for the hospital experience, particularly in connection with surgery' (Mansson *et al.* 1992). This study also revealed that children who did receive psychological preparation reacted in a similar way to those who had received a pre-operative medication alone. The local nursing team came to the conclusion from the literature that psychological preparation was of utmost importance, which led to the establishment of the Saturday Club to give the children the opportunity to find out what would be happening to them when they were admitted to the ward for their surgery.

The variances from the anticipated circumcision Pathway when it was first run, although infrequent were evenly divided between those children who did have a pre-operative medication and those who did not, with no differences in anxiety levels noted between each cohort of children. Thus it appeared that the use of pre-medications had no significant effect on the recovery or anxiety levels of the children concerned.

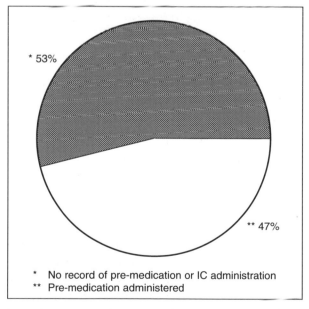

*   53%

**   47%

*   No record of pre-medication or IC administration
** Pre-medication administered

Fig. 7.5   Use of pre-operative medications for children undergoing circumcision.

Armed with this information, the nursing staff met with the anaesthetists and they discussed whether pre-operative medications should be used for all patients, or whether they could be discontinued completely. The team decided that they would stop prescribing pre-medications for all children undergoing this operation, and that anxiety levels would be monitored during the next few months to ensure that it was not contributing to a bad experience for the child and their family. Since this time the unit has shown that despite no pre-operative medication being used, all children are discharged at the expected time, recovering at the same rate, and there has been no increase in the level of anxiety in the children.

Local anaesthetic cream is used to numb the skin when a cannula is inserted for the administration of anaesthesia. The nursing staff were concerned prior to the use of the ICP that a large proportion of the children were not having this cream applied. The ICP stated that each child should have this cream prescribed and applied, and the analysis that followed showed that with the use of this cream specified on the ICP, 97% of cases did then have it prescribed and used (Fig. 7.6). The team is now looking into the prospect of using the ICP as a prescription document for this topical substance, without requiring the doctor to 'write it up' individually for each child on a separate prescription chart.

It is always important to review variances. The analysis of the circumcision cases showed that 83% of them had no variances from the

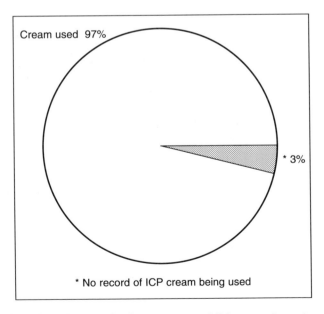

Fig. 7.6 Use of local anaesthetic cream on children undergoing circumcision once its use was specified on the ICP.

Pathway at all. This was not unexpected, as circumcision is a very simple and well co-ordinated procedure with routine processes for recovery. The only variances that occurred (Fig. 7.7) were for post-operative vomiting and swelling of the penis. The figures for these variances were so small that the Pathway was considered to be suitable to continue as it was at that stage.

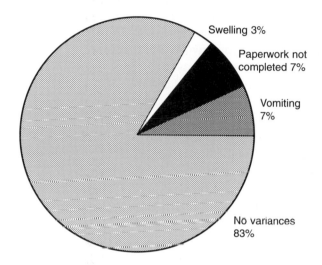

Fig. 7.7   Variances recorded for children undergoing circumcision.

Review of documentation errors enables the team to see how well they are completing the Pathway document, and can act as a reminder to ensure full completion of the document. A small proportion of documentation errors have been identified with each analysis, although the percentage of Pathways with errors or omissions has been below 10% since 1994.

Analysis of the circumcision ICP has continued to take place since the 1994 period. The analyses in 1995 highlighted the need to evaluate variances from the expected condition in the convalescent period after discharge from the ward. To facilitate this, the ICP ensures that before the child goes home with his parents, they are given a contact number for the ward so that if any complications occur once the child is at home, the ward can be informed. The ward staff can then provide advice to the family on what they should do and who they should see. Review of the more medium-term outcomes of surgery beyond the ward setting enables the team to ensure that the care they deliver within the hospital enhances the child's longer term recovery.

Benefits

The benefits of using ICPs affect the child, their family and the clinical staff. For the child, Pathways improve the line of communication between them and the hospital staff. Not only do all members of the multi-disciplinary team know what is to happen and when, but each are able to explain the events of the day to the child. Such explanations to the parents enable them to explain things to their child too. Provision of information and explanations to the child, whether from the Pathway or through the Saturday Club, help to counteract the negative effects of hospitalisation on the child, as admission to hospital is potentially a very frightening experience.

Empowerment of parents, with knowledge of their child's care, can help the parent be more involved in that care and to participate in care delivery when appropriate. Improved lines of communication build stronger relationships between staff and the families, with trust and confidence in the care delivered. Staff thus benefit from calmer, satisfied parents and children.

When agency or locum staff work in the unit, they are not always fully aware of what local best practice is. They too can use the Pathway to inform themselves as to what is to take place each day for the child. Staff also benefit from the provision of planning for discharge right from the first contact with the child, and such planning is co-ordinated by the Pathway. A seamless service can be provided, with outpatient appointments being booked in good time, referrals to support agencies being made at appropriate times in the care, information given to children and their families at the best times in the recovery stages, etc. Criteria for discharge that have been set by the local teams enable the paediatric nurses to take decisions to discharge the child at the stated time on the Pathway, as long as the patient meets all the criteria. As a result far less time is wasted chasing medical teams to review a child and approve their discharge home.

Conclusion

Many other ICPs have since been developed within the paediatric unit, for other surgical procedures and medical conditions too. Lengths of stay have been reduced, teamwork has been improved within the unit, and the provision of information to children and their families has improved markedly too. There is no doubt that ICPs have benefited the unit enormously, helping to create a calmer atmosphere, facilitated through the increased communication between different disciplines and the better co-ordination of care.

References

Brockopp, D.Y., Porter, M., Kinnaird, S. & Sliberman, S. (1992) Fiscal and clinical evaluation of patient care; a case management model for the future. *Journal of Nursing Administration*, **22**, 23–7.

Challinor, J. (1992) The problem with case management. *Journal of Pediatric Nursing*, **7**, 161.

Crummer, M.B. & Carter, V. (1993) Critical Pathways; the Pivotal Tool. *Journal of Cardiovascular Nursing*, **7**, 30–37.

Crummette, B.D. & Boatwright, D.N. (1991) Case management in inpatient pediatric nursing. *Pediatric Nurse*, **17**, 469–73.

Delamothe, T. (1994) Wanted: guidelines that doctors will follow. *British Medical Journal*, **307**, 218.

Maclean, D. (1993) *Clinical Guidelines; A Report to the Scottish Office.* HMSO, London.

Mansson, M., Fredrikson, B. & Rosberg, B. (1992) Comparison of preparation and narcotic-sedative premedication in children undergoing surgery. *Pediatric Nursing*, **18**, (4) 337–42, 350–51.

Parker, D.J. & Cleland, J.G. (1994) Joint audit committee BCS/RCP, London (letter), *British Heart Journal*, **71**, 596.

Schrieffer, J. (1994) The synergy of Pathways and algorithms; two tools are better than one. *Journal of Quality Improvement*, **20**, 485–99.

Shane, R. (1995) Critical Pathways. Take the first step on the critical Pathway. *American Journal of Health System Pharmacology*, **52**, 1051–3.

Turley, K., Tyndall, M., Roge, C., Cooper, M., Turley, K., Applebaum, M. & Tarnoff, H. (1994) Critical Pathway methodology; effectiveness in congenital heart surgery. *Annals of Thoracic Surgery*, **58**, 57–65.

Weingarten, S., Agocs, L., Tankel, N., Sheng, A. & Ellrodt, A.G. (1993) Reducing lengths of stay for patients hospitalised with chest pain using medical practice guidelines and opinion leaders. *American Journal of Cardiology*, **71**, 259–62.

Weinstein, R. (1991) Hospital case management: the path to empower nurses. *Pediatric Nurse*, **17**, 289–93.

Westaby, S. (1994) Cost containment in cardiac surgery: back to basics. NHS Management Executive Value for Money Update, **11**, 4–5.

Acknowledgement

Alison Harper wishes to thank Helen Sibley (link person) for her contribution to the variants analysis.

Chapter 8

Pathways in Accident and Emergency

John Belstead and Karen Thornborrow

Introduction

Accident and emergency medicine is a new speciality of the latter half of this century. It has developed from the old 'casualty departments' which were often the first experience of independent medical practice for the newly qualified doctor. In the days before the British National Health Service (NHS) was conceived in 1948, people who could not afford to pay for family practitioner care were dependent on the local charity or local authority casualty departments for their medical care. Newly qualified doctors were faced with large numbers of patients from the poorer sectors of the community, upon whom they could exercise their newly acquired skills.

As the NHS developed it was recognised that the casualty department was an inappropriate place for the newly qualified to practise, and a requirement was introduced for the doctors within such departments to be fully registered medical practitioners. To be fully registered the junior doctor had to complete one full year as a house officer in a hospital, working under the supervision of a consultant. Today, accident and emergency departments in the UK are still staffed mainly by newly registered doctors who have only been qualified for one year.

Since the 1950s accident and emergency medicine has been recognised as an area of medicine that has sufficient identifiable separate components as to be a speciality in its own right. As this new field of medicine was established, consultant posts were created in 1972 and a training structure developed. Registrar and senior registrar posts were also created. A gradual transition occurred in which the accident and emergency departments left their traditional position of being under the direct control of orthopaedic surgeons, and became independent departments with accident and emergency consultants controlling the medical care within this new speciality.

Now that dedicated specialists are running the accident and emergency departments, they have worked to enhance the service that is provided to the patients attending the units. Training programmes for junior doctors are well established, providing education on the theoretical and practical skills required within this setting of health care delivery. Research and audit have become an integral part of clinical practice within these departments too, enabling review of practices and the evaluation of new treatments and therapies. At the same time politicians, managers and other clinicians have recognised that much of the quality of care provided in a hospital is perceived by the population at large from their experience of the accident and emergency department.

Practitioners of accident and emergency medicine find themselves under increasing scrutiny, with demands to conform to many and often differing standards. Such standards of care can direct clinical care, as with the National Asthma Guidelines issued by the British Thoracic Society *et al.* (1990). Some standards or guidelines require a mixture of clinical and management changes to be achieved, as with trying to achieve a 'door-to-needle time' for thrombolysis administration of 30 minutes. The British government has set up a Patient's Charter (DoH 1992) which has set maximum waiting times and dictated the order of activities within the accident and emergency departments, with the patient being 'triaged' or reviewed by a clinical member of the department team prior to registration at the reception of the unit.

Some of these new developments have been a helpful stimulus to improving the quality of the patient's experience; others have been a tedious and time consuming collection of statistics which may be difficult to analyse in an informative and useful manner.

Developments for improving quality

The first route to increasing the quality of care has been the writing of books for this speciality of medicine. The books have ranged from pocket-sized handbooks to large multi-volume tomes. All authors have struggled with the conflicting priorities of being comprehensive and also being usable on a day to day basis. This has inevitably led to compromises. Some books emphasise the medico-legally important conditions which are seen infrequently but tend to generate negligence litigation, such as the dislocated lunate, or oesophageal rupture. Other books concentrate much more on the injuries and diseases seen on a daily basis, such as simple cuts, sprains, fractures and common acute medical conditions.

Whichever approach is taken by authors, all books have two significant drawbacks within the accident and emergency setting. Firstly, they cannot take into account local traditions and practice; for example, there are a variety of regimens published to calculate fluid replacement in the burned patient, and each of these different regimens is favoured by different burns units or accident and emergency units. Secondly, they suffer from the defect of all books in being slow to update, and therefore it is hard to keep such texts completely up to date with current best practice. This combines with a reluctance on the part of individual doctors and departments to spend large amounts of money on purchasing each new edition of each text as it is published.

With all these difficulties facing them, senior medical staff and departments have adopted a system of booklets of local guidelines and protocols. National guidelines have been published over the years on topics varying from the management of patients with a myocardial infarction (Weston *et al.* 1994), to the management of avulsed teeth (Krasner 1994). Such national guidelines, published by the colleges of medicine and other professional bodies, can be incorporated into a booklet of local guidelines and protocols to be followed within that local unit.

Ashford Hospital NHS Trust, Middlesex, has followed this approach, with each new intake of doctors being given their own copies of such guidelines and protocols. These are produced with each condition summarised on individual A4 sheets, in a loose leaf format, which can be changed and updated frequently and easily, as the understanding of the management of different conditions develops.

There are obvious benefits to this system, yet it has its disadvantages too. Such a booklet of medical guidelines and protocols is very doctor centred. This impedes the development of the multi-disciplinary approach to the care of the acutely ill and injured, which we are trying to establish today. Also these guidelines take a considerable amount of senior medical and secretarial staff time to produce, both initially and whenever they require an update. If these guideline booklets are out of date, they are worse than the old textbooks. Equally, in attempting to keep such documents brief and therefore usable in the clinical situation, they cannot be fully comprehensive, as they must be simple for the doctor to refer to at speed.

Despite the increased profile of the accident and emergency department, very few units in the UK have senior or middle grade medical staff in the unit 24 hours each day. With this situation, appropriate use of relevant and correct guidelines is important to ensure that standards of care are maintained at all times. The difficulty appears to be not the development of such guidelines and protocols of practice, more the way in which these can be integrated directly into clinical practice and patient care at all times. This is where a Pathway, which forms the legal record of patient care and contains all the multi-disciplinary guidelines of practice, is of greatest benefit within an accident and emergency department.

Developing the myocardial infarction Pathway

Within our hospital, the early Integrated Care Pathways (ICPs) were aimed at progressing a patient's stay through the hospital wards, and as such appeared to have little relevance to the very first part of their stay in hospital, in the accident and emergency department. However, the ICP did have the attractive feature of spreading the responsibility for the standard of patient care across the whole multidisciplinary team, with each member of that team having an identified role to play during the patient's episode of care.

Events in the accident and emergency department have a significant effect on the patient's subsequent recovery. For example, many international multi-centre trials have demonstrated the importance of early thrombolysis in myocardial infarction (GISSI 1986; ISIS-2 1988; LATE Study Group 1993). Therefore, care within this department must be prompt and appropriate, without undue delays in the delivery of care and the transfer to a ward, should admission be required. ICPs at Ashford Hospital were therefore extended to include the episode of care in the accident and emergency department, starting with ICPs for fractured neck of femur and myocardial infarction (MI).

In 1992 a regional audit was conducted, and it revealed anticipated wide variations between different hospitals in 'door-to-needle' times for thrombolysis (time from when the patient arrives at the hospital to the time that thrombolysis is administered). Within our hospital itself, we noted differences in the length of stay for these patients within the coronary care unit, and the total number of days spent in hospital. The MI-ICP was developed to cover a patient's care from their arrival in the accident and emergency department, to the time of discharge from hospital.

The first draft of the ICP was ready for pilot by September 1993, following two months spent by a multi-disciplinary team writing it. The team consisted of medical physicians, junior doctors, nurses, cardiac rehabilitation nurse, dietitian, pharmacist and cardiac technicians. The accident and emergency section of the Pathway was written to reflect the critical clinical stages in the diagnosis and treatment of a patient with an MI. A particular emphasis was placed on trying to capture the times of interventions, because of the increasing evidence that time lapse before receiving thrombolysis was a significant factor in the effectiveness of this treatment.

The use of Pathways was a new concept to the staff within the department, so training was needed, both before the ICP was written and once the document was ready to be used. Prior to the use of the Pathway, nurses, doctors and other professionals had maintained physically separate records of the care given to the patient, each of their records structured in a different way despite many items within each record duplicating others. Not surprisingly the most difficult group to get together for the review of records, and the development of the new Pathway document, was the doctors, due to the awkward shift patterns of the casualty officers and the continuous nature of their work whilst on duty.

Implementing the myocardial infarction ICP

Once the MI Pathway was written, training took place for all staff who would be using it in practice. Training included how the document should be completed, explanations on why the Pathway was being used, and how the whole team would receive feedback on the analysis of the Pathway at regular intervals. Training sessions were delivered at different times during the day on many occasions, to ensure that all staff were able to attend.

Once staff were trained, the MI-ICP went 'live', and after the first 30 cases had been cared for on a Pathway the ICPs were analysed to see what variances from the expected care were taking place, and to review the times of thrombolysis delivery. The early version of the Pathway suffered from incomplete entry of data on the document, and variances were not consistently recorded. Investigation as to why this was taking place uncovered resistance from the medical staff to the Pathway and its completion. At this early stage the Pathway did not replace the medical casualty notes, and the doctors were quite understandably reluctant to record data twice – once in the case notes and then again in the Pathway.

The Pathway was then redrafted so that it could function as a medical record, thereby negating the need for separate casualty notes. This resulted in a larger document but one that could be used more readily and was quick to complete. Many of the steps of what is expected to occur in the accident and emergency department for the MI patient is pre-printed on the Pathway, so that the doctor need only fill in times and a signature for each activity. This simpler entry system has enabled a 'fast-track' approach to the care of patients with an MI in this department, avoiding undue delays from the excess of paperwork currently being used in hospitals today (Fig. 8.1).

Nevertheless, resistance from the medical staff is still encountered, primarily due to a mind-set whereby they are only able to see their freehand written notes as valid for a legal record of care. It has been difficult to persuade them to abandon their freehand notes for the simpler ICP, but this will ease with time as the Pathway becomes an accepted and more common form of record keeping.

Results of using the myocardial infarction ICP

Between 1993 and 1996 six analyses of the MI Pathway have taken place, with over 200 individual cases being included. Each time an analysis has been performed, the Pathway has been edited and relaunched. These analyses have given us information on many points, including:

- Length of stay in hospital
- Length of stay in coronary care unit
- Reasons for delays in discharge from hospital
- Reasons for delays in transfer out of coronary care unit
- Percentage of cases admitted to coronary care unit
- Reasons why patients not admitted to coronary care unit
- Co-morbidities associated with MI patients
- Percentage of cases receiving particular drug therapies
- Door-to-needle times for thrombolysis delivery
- Reasons for delayed thombolysis delivery
- Variances from anticipated care
- Percentage of cases referred for cardiac rehabilitation
- Percentage of cases accepting cardiac rehabilitation therapy

During this time we have been able to show improvements in the number of patients admitted to the coronary care unit, through the review of reasons for patients not being admitted there and then appropriate action being taken. We have improved the percentage of cases getting cardiac rehabilitation and those receiving aspirin treatment. Also, the number of patients who receive thrombolysis has increased.

Of greatest importance here is that the Pathway and its analysis enable the team to review care delivery regularly, and pick up on the reasons why things are not always occurring as anticipated. This then provides the opportunity to take action in minimising or eliminating any problems. Equally, the team is able to review new research evidence on care for a particular condition, discuss it, and decide if this evidence should be added to the Pathway and thereby integrated directly into clinical practice.

Benefits

The greatest benefit from the use of a Pathway in the accident and emergency setting is that the Pathway is a consistent method of record keeping which enables the team to have pre-printed guidelines and protocols of care as part of the legal record of care. This permits a consistent approach to the delivery of care between all the different professionals involved in patient care. The team can ensure that consistent best practice is applied at all times, no matter who is on duty.

Paperwork of this kind, that sets out processes for diagnosis and thus aids decision making, encourages fast-track delivery of care, with regular prompts to check contra-indications to suggested treatments like throm-

ACUTE MYOCARDIAL INFARCTION

PATIENT NAME

ON ARRIVAL IN A & E

TIME ARRIVED IN A & E: .... HRS.

Observations: BP .... mmHg   Resps .... per minute

Pulse .... per minute   Temp .... °C

12 lead ECG Recorded [ ]   Cardiac Monitor applied [ ]   Venflon Inserted [ ]

Aspirin 300 mg given   YES [ ]   NO [ ]

If not, why not? _____

EMERGENCY MEDICAL ASSESSMENT

History of present condition   Time of pain onset: .... Hrs.

(IF < 6 hrs. CONSIDER FOR COBALT TRIAL)

CONTRAINDICATIONS TO THROMBOLYSIS

(TICK IF PRESENT)

active bleeding or bleeding diathesis [ ]

history of stroke or CNS structural damage [ ]

major surgery or significant trauma in the past 6 months [ ]

recent non-compressible vascular puncture [ ]

pregnancy, lactation or parturition within the previous 30 days [ ]

and females of childbearing age who are not using adequate birth control

NB: CAUTION IS ADVISED IN PATIENTS WITH UNCONTROLLED HYPERTENSION, defined as a systolic BP of >/= 180mmHg and/or a diastolic BP of >/= 110mmHg in spite of therapy. All efforts should be made to treat the BP effectively before administration of the thrombolytic

IF FOR COBALT TRIAL, COMMENCE COBALT TRIAL PACKAGE

Please tick if on COBALT [ ]

CHOICE OF THROMBOLYTIC: (If not contraindicated)

Tick as appropriate: Streptokinase [ ]

rtPA (to be discussed with PRW) [ ]

If rtPA given - why?   Streptokinase within last 2 years [ ]

Other: (please specify) [ ]

TIME THROMBOLYSIS GIVEN: .... HRS.

Door to needle time : [   ] mins

If door to needle time is > 30 mins, specify reason : ....

RISK FACTORS   Tick if present:-

Smoker ☐
Ex-smoker ☐
Diabetes ☐
Hypertension ☐
Family History ☐
Cholesterol >6.0 ☐

PREVIOUS I.H.D.

Angina ☐
M.I. ☐
CABG / PTCA ☐

DIAGNOSIS

Tick if present: > 2mm ST elevation in 2 or more contiguous chest leads ☐
> 1mm ST elevation in 2 or more limb leads ☐
New left bundle branch block ☐

NB: THERE IS NO EVIDENCE TO SUPPORT THROMBOLYSIS OF
OTHER ECG CHANGES

CARDIAC ENZYMES SHOULD NOT BE MEASURED
IN A/E IN A SUSPECTED ACUTE MI

ANALGESIA
Prescribe & Administer analgesia
(Diamorphine & Metoclopramide I.V.)

Tick if Done ☐

IF THROMBOLYSED (not COBALT)

1/2 hrly BP , P & R maintained for 2 hrs
(recorded on TPR chart)
Cardiac Monitored constantly ☐
Oxygen Saturation monitored constantly ☐

Bed arranged in CCU   yes ☐   If not, why not?
no ☐   No Bed available ☐
Not appropriate for patient ☐
Other ☐

(Please specify) _____

Atenolol 50 mg o.d. prescribed _____
If not, why not? _____

Prescribe 75mg Aspirin o.d. _____

Time transferred from A & E _____ HRS

Transferred to   CCU ☐   Wordsworth ☐   Arnold ☐
Bronte ☐   Keats ☐

or other (please specify) _____

DOCTORS SIGNATURE:

Fig. 8.1   Accident and emergency department section of the MI Pathway from Ashford Hospital NHS Trust.

bolysis. This can be of huge benefit for more junior staff in situations that require quick decisions.

The Pathway also allows referrals to other health care professionals for all patients, and at the most appropriate time in their treatment. Equally, all professionals of whatever discipline, having been involved in the development of the ICP, are then working to identical guidelines and treatment protocols.

With times of treatments also being recorded on the document, more accurate information about interventions and their actual time of administration can be obtained, with delays being picked up with ease and accounted for. This gives us the added benefit of providing in-built audit of care and the speed of that care, which provides data for the purchasers of health care without the department having to carry out an independent audit that can be very time consuming and complicated. Such audit is also prospective rather than the more traditional retrospective audits of the past.

The doctors do not only benefit from the simple paperwork and continuous audit of multi-disciplinary care; they are also able to follow the treatment patterns without an acclimatisation period when new to the unit. This means that locum staff are able to follow the protocols that the department prefers by using the document.

Other ICPs in the accident and emergency department

As already mentioned, we have developed an ICP for the care of the fractured neck of femur patient within the department. This ICP has enabled us to monitor how long it takes to get our patients to theatre from admission to the unit, and through this review more cases are now being operated upon on the same day as admission.

Other Pathways include an asthma Pathway. The development of this Pathway has illustrated the need for care in designing an ICP, and the problems that can arise. A single protocol sheet was produced for use by the junior doctors within the department. The difficulty was to get that document referred to and used for every patient attending the department with an asthma attack. The document tended to be used for patients with the most severe exacerbations, and not for those with a mild attack but who were still in need of expeditious and appropriate treatment.

The Pathway was written based on the British Thoracic Society's (1990) guidelines, and its final appearance was somewhat similar to the original protocol sheet but was found to be more difficult to follow by the junior doctors. This highlights the need for every Pathway, once written, to be piloted; until it has been tried out in the real setting you cannot be sure that it is entirely usable. The asthma Pathway is being rewritten ready for a relaunch soon. This is the nature of Pathways; they are dynamic documents that need to be constantly upgraded and edited to ensure that they are always user-friendly for the staff who will be completing them, as well as being up to date.

More Pathways are being developed all the time, predominantly for the most common conditions that are admitted to hospital through the accident and emergency department.

Conclusion

Pathways have much to offer the accident and emergency department. They have the advantage of being developed locally, making them both relevant and relatively easily updated. This does not mean that generally accepted national or international standards, or guidelines of care are ignored; these guidelines can be readily incorporated into the Pathway. Being produced locally, however, the Pathways are more likely to obtain local acceptance and ownership. It is essential that all the staff in a hospital can see the documents as relevant for them, and that their input into the development process is valued. This would not be achieved from an externally imposed document.

Embarking on a process of implementing Pathways is not something to be undertaken lightly. They cannot simply be produced and left to run. Their strength lies in the process of continuous review and the analysis of variances. If this is not done, they are merely a glorified guideline. The process of developing, analysing and modifying a Pathway requires commitment from the clinical team and the support of an individual whose principal task is to work with the clinical team in this process. Such a person will need to be enthusiastic and able to use a computer for document production and analysis. Above all, they will need to be able to enthuse managers, nurses, therapists and, most difficult of all, senior medical staff, because they will all need to commit time to this process for the benefit of their patients.

References

British Thoracic Society, Research Unit of the Royal College of Physicians, Kings Fund Centre, National Asthma Campaign (1990) Guidelines for management of asthma in adults. *British Medical Journal*, **301**, 6 October, 797–800.

DoH (1992) *The Patient's Charter*. HMSO, London.

GISSI (1986) Gruppo Italiano per lo Studio della Steptochinasi nell'Infarto miocardico: Effectiveness of Intravenous Thrombolytic Treatment in Acute Myocardial Infarction. *Lancet*, **1**, 397–402.

ISIS-2 (1988) Second international study of infarct survival: randomized trial of intravenous streptokinase, oral aspirin, both, or neither among 17,187 cases of suspected myocardial infarction. *Lancet*, **II**, 349–60.

Krasner, P. (1994) Modern treatment of avulsed teeth by emergency physicians. *American Journal of Emergency Medicine*, **12**(2) 241–6.

LATE Study Group (1993) Late assessment of thrombolytic efficacy study with alteplase 6–24 hours after onset of acute myocardial infarction. *Lancet*, **342**, 759–66.

Weston, C.F., Penny, W.J. & Julian, D.G. (1994) Guidelines for the early management of patients with myocardial infarction. *British Medical Journal*, **308**, 767–71.

Part 3

Pathways in the Non-acute Setting

Chapter 9

Pathways Bridging the Acute/Community Interface

Ann Higginson and Sue Johnson

Introduction

The trend towards the provision of home care rather than extended hospital stays has been very gradual in Britain. 'Hospital at Home', however, has been in existence in Europe and America since the 1960s. The idea for Hospital at Home originated in France and was first established in 1961 in the Paris suburb of Bayonne. This original scheme provided a home care service for patients suffering from cancer.

It was not until 1972 that this concept of care delivery came to England following a visit to France by Freda Clark, a senior social worker, whilst studying community care options. After discussions with the Department of Health and Social Security a similar scheme was established some seven years later in Peterborough. This first British scheme was funded from the Sainsbury Trust (a charitable organisation), with Peterborough being chosen because of its rapidly growing population which was, in part, out-stripping the acute hospital facilities. It is interesting to note that although the Peterborough Hospital at Home scheme commenced in 1979, it was not until the late 1980s and early 1990s that other similar projects were initiated in this country, and most of these tended to be based in rural areas.

The Tomlinson Report (1992) highlighted the need for a shift of resources from secondary to primary care. Together with the rapidly changing scientific and technological advances, changes in illness patterns, improved sanitation and demographic trends, the recommendations of this report led to a number of Tomlinson funded Hospital at Home schemes being implemented in the London area.

A major problem facing both health and social service resources is the steadily increasing numbers of older people, particularly over the age of 80. Increases in population age have an impact on the occurrence of multiple pathology, particularly in those illnesses associated with old age: fractured neck of femur, cerebral vascular accident, chest and heart diseases. Mental confusional states also pose a considerable problem both for the management of these patients in an acute facility, and for providing comprehensive packages of care for them in their own homes. There is now much evidence to suggest that older patients who remain in hospital are more likely to end up in institutions or gain a hospital acquired infection or complication; it can thus be argued that early discharge home from hospital will provide better outcomes than if the patient remains longer in hospital.

Concerns are also being raised about the overall costs of inpatient care, and Hospital at Home is considered possibly a cheaper option to acute care; however, no in-depth financial comparison has yet been completed. A costing exercise was undertaken on the orthopaedic project within the Peterborough scheme, although this is a 'rural' scheme which can work with more 'bank' staffing systems, which allows financial savings. Within the London projects, due to the lack of availability of staff to work on a 'bank' or 'work when required' basis, such savings have not been available, resulting in multi-disciplinary teams being employed for the duration of each project.

It is probable that Hospital at Home will not produce the large amounts of savings predicted for the following reasons:

- Considerable expense is incurred through staff travelling costs
- Many London projects are funded for the short term only; long term funding would require hospital beds to be closed to enable transfer of funds
- Closing acute beds would only save direct staff costs, not the indirect or overhead costs
- With patients going into Hospital at Home schemes, the dependency of patients left in hospital would rise, with the acute units requiring higher levels of skilled staff

Activity would inevitably rise in the acute facilities if patients were transferred back to their own homes for convalescence, or the less complicated conditions remained at home. With elective surgery patients being discharged home earlier, the throughput of such patients would also increase, impacting on activity levels.

Establishing a Hospital at Home service is not always an easy task, and there are many concerns from all disciplines involved, including:

- The potential increase in workload for general practitioners and district nurses
- The reluctance on the part of hospital based staff to co-operate due to the implications for potential bed reductions to secure long term funding
- The ability of some community based staff to provide the care required for more acute patients than were previously cared for in the community setting

- Schemes of this type are seen as a cost cutting exercise and not as an improvement in service to the patient through a more qualitative approach to individualised patient care

One final comment in this introduction to Hospital at Home schemes is the impact of such a method of care delivery upon the 'informal carers' or families of the patients. For them there is likely to be a cost, both in financial terms and in the pressure on their time. The impact of Hospital at Home on such carers has yet to be evaluated.

Hospital at Home in Hounslow and Spelthorne

The Hounslow and Spelthorne Hospital at Home scheme received Tomlinson funding of £280 000 per year for two and a half years from April 1994. This project aims to provide hospital level care to adult patients in the comfort of their own home.

A project manager was appointed in January 1994 and a multi-disciplinary/multi-agency steering group was established. Members of this group included health, social and voluntary agencies as well as a representative from the Community Health Council and Carers National. A project management team was also set up, again representing the many disciplines and agencies, to produce the policies, procedures and protocols required for the management of the project and service. This project is being formally evaluated by the Kensington, Chelsea and Westminster Public Health Department for cost and quality of service.

The Integrated Care Pathway (ICP) co-ordinators from the two local acute hospitals linked with the scheme were appointed to both the steering group and project management team, as Pathways were seen as the tool for enabling continuity of patient care across the acute/community interface, whilst providing a framework of practice for all disciplines of health care workers involved in the delivery of care. Equally, the Pathway system offered an audit tool for the continuous review of the care delivered.

During the six months before patients were accepted onto the scheme, time was spent by the project manager meeting staff of all disciplines, both in the acute facilities and in the community, and talking with the other agencies. This was to build up strong relationships with the services already provided within the area, so that all agencies could work together for the improvement of the patient's experience. The project manager also investigated existing schemes throughout the country to learn from their experiences, whilst also linking with Hospital at Home projects throughout London to see where these individual projects could interface.

The Hospital at Home core team was made up of two nurse practitioners, senior physiotherapy and occupational therapy staff and health care assistants. This team worked very closely with the ICP co-ordinators to set up the Pathways for orthopaedic cases.

Developing the Pathways

The Hospital at Home scheme offers the patient the choice of being cared for in their own home, rather than staying in hospital. The project began with elective orthopaedic patients for the development of the initial Pathways. The process for a patient coming onto the Hospital at Home scheme was:

- Patient attends the orthopaedic pre-admission clinic one week prior to admission, where the concept of Hospital at Home is introduced and the Pathway of Care explained
- Consent from the patient, their key carer, surgical consultant and general practitioner obtained
- Hospital at Home team visits patient at home, prior to admission, to assess the suitability of their home for inclusion in the scheme
- Patient admitted for surgery
- Patient transferred home early into Hospital at Home care
- Patient's care completed in their own home, until discharge from care

The Pathways written were for total hip replacement (THR) and total knee replacement (TKR). The acute hospital at Ashford already had inpatient Pathways for these procedures, so a team of acute and community staff was convened for two meetings, to adapt the acute Pathway to accommodate the early transfer home for some patients.

Two separate Pathways were developed: one was the original inpatient ICP for those patients who did not go onto the Hospital at Home scheme, and the second was a similar Pathway for Hospital at Home patients. Both forms of ICPs covered the pre-admission clinic and ran until the patient was either discharged from hospital, for ordinary patients, or discharged from the Hospital at Home scheme, for the project's patients (Fig. 9.1).

Before the Pathways could be implemented, a pilot phase was needed to test out the content of the Pathway documents and the practicalities of the process. Transferring post-operative hospital care into the community setting required aspects of care on the Pathway to be adjusted to accommodate the facilities and assessments performed in the community (Fig. 9.2).

Difficulties were expected as the acute staff understood the process of mapping care with a Pathway, but did not fully comprehend care delivery issues within the community setting; conversely the community staff, who

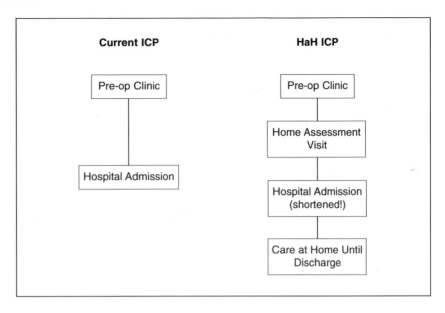

Fig. 9.1   Inpatient ICP and Hospital at Home ICP care routes.

understood care within their setting, did not fully comprehend the Pathway process at first and found it hard to map care. Nursing documentation in the community has been upgraded during the past ten years, and the district nursing staff were not keen at this time to change their paperwork once more, and were very suspicious at the reduction in the amount of record keeping needed with the ICP system.

Much training was required for all community staff on the use of the ICP document, particularly on how to complete variances. There were many problems with accessibility to the community staff; they were working over wide geographical areas, with large caseloads. Organised training sessions were not well attended, which hindered the successful use of the document once the ICPs went live. This issue required further attention when the pilot developed into a full implementation of Pathways.

Implementing the pathways

A date was set and the pilot commenced, with every patient then attending the orthopaedic pre-admission clinic which was being offered Hospital at Home. The choice of Pathway (ordinary inpatient or Hospital at Home) was dependent upon the choice made by the patient. This seemed to be a great way of commencing the correct Pathway document prior to the pilot, yet at

INTEGRATED CARE PATHWAY
HOSPITAL AT HOME
Total Hip Replacement

Patient Name: ....

	PRE-OP CLINIC Date:	HOME ASSESSMENT Date:	DAY 1 ADMISSION Date:	DAY 2 OPERATION DAY Date: .... PRE - OP WARD
CLINICAL ASSESSMENT	DOCTORS CLERKING OPERATION EXPLAINED CONSENT SIGNED 3M SCORE COMPLETED NURSING ASSESSMENT (to include) BLOOD PRESSURE WEIGHT URINALYSIS MEASURE FOR TEDs AND RECORD ON FRONT SHEET PHYSIOTHERAPY ASSESSMENT	ACCOMODATION ASSESSED ACCORDING TO CRITERIA ALL CRITERIA MET FOR INCLUSION ON HAH SCHEME	NOTES AVAILABLE BLOOD RESULTS AVAILABLE X-RAY AVAILABLE BASELINE TPR BP RECORDED SEEN BY ANAESTHETIST IODINE SENSITIVITY TEST PERFORMED NAMEBAND AND ALLERGY BAND (if req) APPLIED REPEAT URINALYSIS PERFORMED WATERLOW SCORE RECORDED	COMMENCE FLUID CHART SURGICAL SITE MARKED BY DOCTOR CHECK CONSENT FORM
TREATMENT	PROPOSED PROSTHESIS :			APPLY TED STOCKINGS CLEAN GOWN AND LINEN SEND TO THEATRE ON BED WITH MULLER SPLINT
REFERRALS	REFER TO SOCIAL WORKER Y IF NECESSARY N			
MEDICATION/ IVs	PREPARE DRUG CHART		CLEXANE GIVEN 12 HOURS PRIOR TO SURGERY	PRE - MED GIVEN 1 HOUR PRE - OP
DIET	EXPLAIN AND ADVISE TO EAT HIGH FIBRE DIET	EXPLAIN AND ADVISE TO EAT HIGH FIBRE DIET	HIGH FIBRE	NBM 6 HOURS PRE - OP

ACTIVITY		COMMENCE DISTRICT NURSE DOCUMENTATION	PRACTISE BREATHING AND LEG EXERCISES	BATH
TEACHING / PSYCHOSOCIAL	EXPLAIN ICP	EXPLAIN HAH SCHEME IN DETAIL	ORIENTATE TO WARD ENVIRONMENT	REASSURE
	HAH SCHEME EXPLAINED	ASSESS FOR UNDERSTANDING	DISCUSS HIP LEAFLET WITH PATIENT	
	HIP INFORMATION LEAFLET GIVEN TO PATIENT	PROVIDE OPPORTUNITY FOR QUESTIONS	RE EXPLAIN ICP AND CHECK UNDERSTANDING	
	ADVICE GIVEN RE ITEMS TO BRING INTO HOSPITAL		EXPLAIN PCA	
DISCHARGE PLAN	DISCUSS EXPECTED DATE OF DISCHARGE	ASSESS EXPECTED NEEDS ON TRANSFER HOME FROM HOSPITAL	CONFIRM EXPECTED DISCHARGE DATE WITH PATIENT	
	DISCUSS POTENTIAL NEEDS ON DISCHARGE WITH PATIENT	COMPLETE EVALUATION QUESTIONNAIRE		
RADIOLOGY / OTHER	CHEST X - RAY			
	PELVIC X - RAY			
	ECG			
LABORATORY	FULL BLOOD COUNT			
	E.S.R.			
	U & Es			
	GROUP AND SCREEN 3 UNITS OF BLOOD			

Fig. 9.2   1994 ICP for a total hip replacement patient on the Hospital at Home scheme.

INTEGRATED CARE PATHWAY

Total Hip Arthroplasty

Patient Name: _____

	POST-OP / WARD DATE:	DAY 3 / 1ST POD DATE:	DAY 4 / 2ND POD DATE:	DAY 5 / 3RD POD DATE:	DAY 6 / 4TH POD DATE:
MEDICAL & NURSING ASSESSMENT	TPR & BP RECORDED HALF HOURLY FOR 2 HOURS; REDIVACS PATENT; REDIVACS MARKED AT MIDNIGHT; PAIN ASSESSMENT PERFORMED; NAUSEA/VOMITING CONTROLLED; REASSESS WATERLOW SCORE AND RECORD; CHECK SPECIAL POST-OP INSTRUCTIONS	ASSESS PRESSURE AREAS; ENSURE REDIVACS PATENT; 4 HOURLY TPR & BP; PAIN ASSESSMENT PERFORMED; NO FRESH BLEEDING ON WOUND; PASSING URINE FREELY	ASSESS PRESSURE AREAS; B.D. T & P; PAIN ASSESSED; WOUND ASSESSED	ASSESS PRESSURE AREAS; B.D. T & P; PAIN ASSESSED; WOUND ASSESSED FOR SIGNS OF INFECTION	ASSESS PRESSURE AREAS; B.D. T & P; PAIN ASSESSED; WOUND ASSESSED FOR SIGNS OF INFECTION; PATIENT NOT CONSTIPATED
TREATMENTS		STOP FLUID CHART	REMOVE REDIVACS; LEAVE SUTURE LINE EXPOSED; DRESS DRAIN SITES	DRESS DRAIN SITES; MR. WALSH PATIENTS:- TRIM ENDS OF DISSOLVING SUTURES	EXPOSE DRAIN SITES
REFERRALS					REFER TO OT (IF NEEDED)
MEDICATION	ANTI-EMETICS GIVEN IF REQUIRED; CEFUROXIME IV X 2 DOSES GIVEN; CLEXANE S/C GIVEN A.M. P.M.	PCA DISCONTINUED; ORAL ANALGESIA COMMENCED; CLEXANE S/C GIVEN A.M. P.M.	CLEXANE S/C GIVEN A.M. P.M.	PRESCRIBE TTA'S; COLLECT TTA'S; CLEXANE S/C GIVEN A.M. P.M.	CLEXANE S/C GIVEN A.M. P.M.
IVIs	BLOOD - 2 UNITS GIVEN; FLUIDS - 1 UNIT GIVEN	DISCONTINUE IVI	REMOVE VENFLON		

PATIENT ACTIVITY	ASSIST TO SIT UP 45° WHEN AWAKE LIFT HEELS FREE OF BED HOURLY	WASH IN BED NURSE WASH BACK & BOTTOM BREATHING & LEG EXERCISES ASSIST HIP EXERCISES IN BED PHYSIO TO SIT PATIENT IN UPRIGHT CHAIR.	WASH IN CHAIR NURSE WASH BACK & BOTTOM WASH LEGS & REAPPLY TEDS HIP EXERCISES IN BED INCREASE MOBILISING & GAIT WITH ZIMMER FRAME	WASH IN CHAIR WALK UP & DOWN WARD WITH ZIMMER FRAME PERFORM BED EXERCISES ALONE	WASH IN BATHROOM WALKING AROUND WARD WITH FRAME INDEPENDENTLY (E.G. TO TOILET AND TO TABLE FOR MEALS)
DIET	NBM UNTIL AWAKE	HIGH FIBRE	HIGH FIBRE	HIGH FIBRE	HIGH FIBRE
DISCHARGE PLANNING	COMPLETE PROSTHESIS CARD			BOOK OPD 6/52 ARRANGE TRANSPORT HOME	GP / NURSE LETTER WRITTEN, REGARDING REMOVAL OF STITCHES ON 12TH POD
TEACHING PSYCHOSOCIAL SUPPORT		REINFORCE TEACHING	REINFORCE TEACHING	REINFORCE TEACHING	REINFORCE TEACHING
RADIOLOGY/ OTHER		CHECK X - RAY			
LABORATORY			CHECK HB		

Fig. 9.2 *continued.*

PATIENT NAME: ....

INTEGRATED CARE PATHWAY (HOSPITAL AT HOME)

Total Hip Replacement

	5th POD — WARD	TRANSFER HOME — HOME	6th POD	7th POD	8th POD
	Date:		Date:	Date:	Date:
CLINICAL ASSESSMENT	ASSESS PRESSURE AREAS BD T P R BP ASSESS CRITERIA FOR TRANSFER : NO INFECTION NO SIGNS OF DVT PAIN CONTROLLED MOBILE WITH FRAME ALL CRITERIA FOR TRANSFER MET	FULL ASSESSMENT TO INCLUDE: WATERLOW SCORE TPR BP LIFTING ASSESSMENT COMMENCE PATIENT PAIN SELF-ASSESSMENT SCORE	ASSESS WOUND REVIEW PATIENT'S PAIN SCORE BD T P R BP	ASSESS WOUND REVIEW PATIENT'S PAIN SCORE BD T P R BP	ASSESS WOUND REVIEW PATIENTS PAIN SCORE BD T P R BP ASSESS CRITERIA FOR DISCHARGE FROM SCHEME: MOBILE WITH STICKS NO INFECTION NO SIGNS OF DVT PAIN CONTROLLED CRITERIA FOR DISCHARGE MET
TREATMENTS					
REFERRALS					
MEDICATIONS					
ACTIVITY	WASH AND DRESS INDEPENDENTLY MOBILISE WITH FRAME	INDEPENDENT WITH FRAME	INDEPENDENT WITH FRAME WASH AND DRESS INDEPENDENTLY	TRANSFER TO STICKS CLIMB STAIRS WITH SUPERVISION WASH AND DRESS INDEPENDENTLY	INDEPENDENT WITH STICKS SAFE ON STAIRS WITH STICKS WASH AND DRESS INDEPENDENTLY

DIET	HIGH FIBRE		HIGH FIBRE		HIGH FIBRE		HIGH FIBRE		HIGH FIBRE
LABORATORY									
RADIOLOGY/ OTHER									
TEACHING/ SUPPORT	EXPLAIN TTA's	REVIEW HOSPITAL DISCHARGE ADVICE WITH PATIENT AND CARER(S)		CHECK THAT PATIENT UNDERSTANDS THE HIP LEAFLET					
DISCHARGE PLAN	GIVE TTA's GIVE OPD **TRANSFER HOME**	COMPLETE EVALUATION QUESTIONNAIRE						**DISCHARGE FROM SCHEME** INFORM GP OF DISCHARGE GIVE CONTACT NUMBERS	

Fig. 9.2 *continued.*

VARIANCE TRACKING SHEET

Total Hip Arthroplasty

WARD _____

Patient Name _____

DATE	DAY NO	TIME	VARIANCE & REASON FOR IT	VARIANCE CODE	ACTION TAKEN	SIGNATURE

PATIENT CONDITION

1	PYREXIA
2	WOUND OOZING/BLEEDING
3	WOUND INFECTED
4	REDIVAC SITE OOZING
5	DISLOCATION
6	URINE RETENTION
7	PAIN NOT CONTROLLED
8	NAUSEA & VOMITING
8A	LOW Hb/ANAEMIA
8B	CONSTIPATED
8C	MOBILITY DIFFICULTIES
8D	PRESSURE SORES
9	OTHER

STAFF/PERSONS

10	FAMILY NOT AVAILABLE
11	DOCTOR DECISION
12	DOCTOR AVAILABILITY
13	NURSE DECISION
14	NURSE AVAILABILITY
14a	PHYSIO DECISION
14b	PHYSIO AVAILABILITY
14c	OT DECISION
14d	OT AVAILABILITY

DEPARTMENTS/SYSTEM

15	PHYSIO CLOSED (BH/WE)
16	OT CLOSED (BH/WE)
17	PHARMACY DELAY
18	TRANSPORT DELAY
19	LABS DELAY
20	X-RAY DELAY
21	COMMUNITY CARE DELAY
22	BED AVAILABILITY
23	EQUIPMENT AVAILABILITY
24	HOME VISIT REQUIRED

Fig. 9.2 *continued.*

this clinic the Hospital at Home team were unable to gain general practitioner and key carer consent for that patient coming onto the scheme, and hence the orthopaedic teams were unable to start the patients on the Hospital at Home ICP at this stage. Thus every patient for THR or TKR attending this clinic was commenced on the inpatient ICPs.

This had little effect on the inpatient care of the patient, as the Pathway still mapped out expected care and co-ordinated the efforts of the acute hospital teams. However, the acute Pathway did not have the facility to continue with the patient back in their own home, as the Hospital at Home Pathways would have done. In this way, the pilot for Hospital at Home Pathways effectively failed, preventing the community teams from having any audit data with which to review their practices as intended.

A meeting with both acute and community staff demonstrated that the failure was in the make-up of the document. One single Pathway document that follows the patient out of the acute hospital and into their own home was impractical and unworkable for this area. The team redesigned the format of the document to have two parallel Pathways, one for the acute setting (pre-admission clinic and inpatient stay), and one for the community setting (pre-admission home visit and care at home after transfer from hospital). In this way the ICP could still be commenced at the pre-admission clinic stage, and it did not then matter if the patient went on the Hospital at Home scheme or not, as the same ICP document applied for the pre-admission clinic and the corresponding inpatient episode (Fig. 9.3). It was set up so that the patient could be transferred home early with Hospital at Home on the third to eighth post-operative day, with their care effectively 'dropping' into the corresponding third to eighth post-operative day on the community ICP. If the patient was not eligible for the Hospital at Home scheme, their episode of care was completed in hospital, co-ordinated by the inpatient ICP until discharge.

With these two parallel ICP documents, it has made it much clearer who is responsible for the completion of the community and acute Pathways. Ownership of the documents by the acute and community teams has also improved. The teams for developing these Pathways have been large, yet this simply reflects the large numbers of staff and disciplines involved in the whole episode of care for elective surgery, both from primary and secondary care. Keeping the authoring teams small would have made acceptance of the document by all staff members difficult, therefore the effort in facilitating large teams was worth the investment.

Three ICPs are now in use for orthopaedic Hospital at Home cases: for THR and TKR as before, and now for fractured neck of femur when the Pathway document commences in the accident and emergency setting.

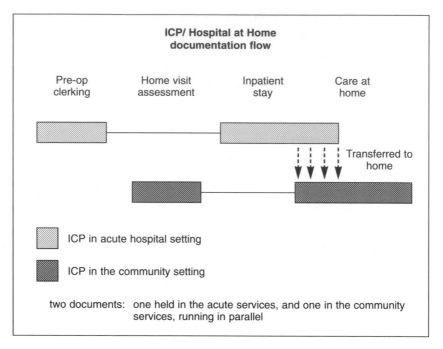

Fig. 9.3   Parallel ICPs for the hospital and community staff.

Results

Analysis of the inpatient Pathways has been taking place for some years, and since the introduction of the Hospital at Home scheme changes have been demonstrated for the lengths of stay. Even though the Pathways did not actually continue in the patient's own home in the early stages of the project, the ICPs were co-ordinating the inpatient care, and the Hospital at Home cases were being transferred home from as early as three days post-operation.

For the TKR patients, the median average length of stay had been reduced by five days with the introduction of the ICPs for inpatient care. Once the Hospital at Home scheme got underway, this reduced by a further two days; this was with fewer than 25% of TKR cases being transferred onto the Hospital at Home scheme. Dividing the lengths of stay for Hospital at Home and non-Hospital at Home cases, the median averages were 6.5 days (Hospital at Home) and 10 days (non-Hospital at home). This suggests that the provision of Hospital at Home has had a significant impact on the length of hospital stay for these elective cases.

Recent figures show that the number of patients entering the Hospital at Home scheme is increasing, which should lead to a positive impact on the availability of beds in the acute setting. Yet, as indicated in the introduction, with elective cases being transferred home early in their recovery phase, and then more patients being admitted for surgery, the dependency of patients on the orthopaedic ward will increase tremendously, thereby putting more pressure on the nursing and therapy staff from greatly increased workloads; this should be considered when reviewing staffing levels and skill-mix within the acute units.

With the introduction of the new parallel system of Pathway documents, a community ICP co-ordinator, together with the acute ICP co-ordinator, is to perform analysis on both sets of completed Pathways, and then outcomes of care may be compared for the two routes of care delivery.

Evaluation of satisfaction with the Hospital at Home scheme has been performed, with questionnaires to both the patients and their key carers. Results from these evaluations have been extremely positive. The following are some of the comments:

- 'Every part of your scheme is excellent – many thanks'
- 'I loved the fact that I could be in my own home'
- 'The care assistants were excellent in helping me with my general needs and were flexible with arrangements'
- 'The assistants worked together so well and at no time was I let down; each one was so efficient and capable; I was very impressed'
- 'I think the staff did an excellent job helping my mother'.

Benefits

The Hospital at Home scheme using the Pathways covers the care and treatments that the patient receives from pre-admission through to discharge from community care. In order that quality care may be provided throughout, the processes of service delivery must be well co-ordinated between the acute hospitals and the community. Pathways help to provide such co-ordination. The Pathway draws together all the different components and activities that will occur throughout the whole clinical episode onto one set of documentation. With this, all staff (acute and community based) will know what care and treatments are to be serviced and they can also see what has taken place before their contact with the patient.

ICPs within a scheme that interfaces the acute and community settings help to provide seamless care through much improved co-ordination. The communication between the settings is easier and improved. Staff from each setting obtain better understanding of each other's roles and functions, and hence work towards improving the interface further. Pathways also offer a facility by which the whole episode of care may be continuously audited for all clinical disciplines involved in care. This in turn promotes service and practice review, with the opportunity to monitor clinical outcomes.

The final benefit of the use of Pathways is to the patient. With the ICP, staff can be sure that all required information and explanation of care and treatments is given to the patient. The patient can follow the ICP day by day, keeping them up to date on their progress and enabling them to ask questions when they wish. The Pathway provides clear information for the patient on their expected care, together with explanations for any variances in care that may occur. Information for patients is an important aspect of patient care in today's health service, and the Pathway can ensure that this service is provided.

Conclusion

Pathways of Care have a significant role to play in the co-ordination of care, which has particular impact on providing a seamless service between the secondary and primary sectors. Although Pathways have only recently been successfully used within the Hounslow and Spelthorne Hospital at Home scheme, many lessons have been learnt from the pilot run about what is practical, feasible and yet useful. We have discovered that a single Pathway document is not practical within our local setting; setting a date of transfer home is not always feasible and the Pathway must be more flexible. Finally, the Pathway is of much more use if it can replace much of the existing paperwork.

Pathways are harder to set up for a broader span of care, particularly when it traverses several care settings, yet the investment in time and effort is worthwhile due to the benefits gained from the process.

Reference

Tomlinson, B. (1992) *Report of the Inquiry into London's Health Service, Medical Education and Research*. HMSO, London.

Chapter 10

Pathways in Community Mental Health

Jenny Thornton

Introduction

'You can't write Anticipated Recovery Pathways for community based services because each patient is an individual with a unique set of needs.' This was, and still is in many professional forums, the cry that goes up when the subject of Pathways of Care is raised in relation to community health care provision.

The arguments at first seem very reasonable. Much of the recent NHS legislation lays emphasis on providing flexible services which are responsive to the individual's needs and preferences and which offer choice. One of the hallmarks of community based services is that they are delivered by several members of the multi-disciplinary team. Not only are these professionals from a wide range of clinical backgrounds, but often from a number of different agencies. This demands collaboration and co-operation from a group of individuals from varied backgrounds with regard to training, skills and, often most significantly, different philosophies of care. How then can we hope to sketch an Anticipated Recovery Pathway (ARP) for any client group cared for in the community?

Unlike clients admitted to hospitals, clients in the community will usually not be aiming for 'recovery'. Community services are often targeted to prevent admission to hospital, reduce the need for extended periods of inpatient stays, enhance the quality of life for individuals and families or carers, and allow individuals to achieve their potential for a healthy life in the community. Care may be 'continuous' over an entire lifetime as each individual requires services to be provided to meet his or her particular needs within a unique home life. How then can anyone hope to write a Pathway for each episode of care? Surely it is unrealistic?

It is for many of these very real reasons that audit, evaluation and research in the community have been limited, piecemeal, patchy and inconclusive to date. Very few interventions currently offered within the community can boast a sound grounding in research or demonstrate proven or even tested outcomes. But does this scepticism really stand up under careful scrutiny? New legislation and guidelines are urging us to commit more resources to community based provision of health care, so we should be examining current practice to establish which interventions give us good outcomes and which fail to achieve their aims.

How can we begin to demonstrate the effectiveness of work in the community? How can we challenge established practice which does not appear to produce good outcomes? More specifically, what are the aims of our services? Do we need such highly qualified and skilled practitioners in the field, and if so, are we training enough of them? If the general public are presented with a new intervention on the television which is reported to 'work miracles', how can we then defend established practice in this country? If our purchasers move towards 'evidence based contracting', how will we support and ideally drive the process as providers of the service?

Developing the Pathways

The issues described in the introduction were some of those facing the Hounslow and Spelthorne Community and Mental Health NHS Trust in the early 1990s. Added to this were the demands by the local purchasers of health care for evaluation of the services we were providing. A visit from the regional Anticipated Recovery Pathway (ARP) group could not have been more timely. With a minor change in the title, here were the answers to our questions: Integrated Care Pathways (ICPs). Rather than attempting to describe the Pathway to recovery suggested by the term 'Anticipated Recovery Pathway', we could instead focus on defining patient groups and setting out our procedures and protocols in a way which described our 'approach' to the care of these client groups.

In the winter of 1993, the Hounslow and Spelthorne Community and Mental Health NHS Trust authorised the author and the lead clinician for child and adolescent psychiatry services to take the Integrated Care Pathway concept back to the department of child and adolescent psychiatry to discuss the piloting of a community mental health ICP. Not only was this to be the first community ICP, but it was also within the field of mental health, another area in which the arguments against the use of Pathways were strong.

A brief synopsis of the history of the department of child and adolescent psychiatry in Hounslow and Spelthorne is necessary at this stage, for the reader to appreciate fully the tangled web of politics and conflicting procedures that existed around the time of the introduction of the first ICP.

In 1990 there were three consultant child psychiatrists working across

Hounslow and Spelthorne, West London. Each of the consultants led a department with quite separate policies and procedures and markedly different approaches to care. Less than one year later, one consultant had retired, a new consultant had been appointed, two general offices had been amalgamated and the main department had been relocated to a base in the community away from the original hospital site.

One of the critical elements of a successful and smooth-functioning multi-disciplinary team is the administrative support, and the most disruptive change to the department had been the necessary amalgamation of the two secretarial teams. The staff were grappling with the impossible task of providing an efficient service to a newly formed and rather unsettled clinical department. There were differences of opinion within both the administrative and clinical teams as to which procedures should take precedence in the new department, and difficulties arose when it came to establishing new roles and relationships.

This was the unsettled environment into which ICPs were introduced. The project team, consisting initially of the care group manager (author) and the consultant lead clinician, decided that an administrative Pathway should be set up from the time that a family was first referred to the department to the point of allocation to a clinician.

The process of setting up an administrative Pathway

With the decision made to set up an ICP, it was time to put the concept to the administrative team. A member of the regional ARP team visited to talk to the group about Pathways, their history, benefits, and structure.

Discussions then took place involving all members of the department's clinical and administrative staff. Taking into account the fragile environment due to the recent changes, it was decided to involve every member of the administrative team in the writing of the Pathway. The first meeting of the full administrative team, with the author as facilitator, was set up and within minutes of sitting down to document the process there was heated debate. At what point should the Pathway really start? Was a verbal referral counted or should it be received in writing before it was recorded?

It was becoming increasingly clear that there was more at stake here for the individuals than the mere writing of a Pathway or the describing of current practices and procedures. We were observing the realities of team working, or rather the absence of it! There quickly emerged two main sides to the discussions, each defending the two sets of procedures brought from each original department. New roles were being tested and relationships were quickly becoming strained.

During the months following the amalgamation of the two departments, the secretaries had been providing what appeared to be one unified service; in reality they had functioned in spite of the changes, choosing not to openly challenge the differences in their procedures. In many cases it became clear that the differences had not been identified. The two teams effectively worked around the differences, providing two separate services each with widely differing standards, stationery and procedures. It was less disruptive and painful to avoid the issues than to address and resolve them.

Only when the time came to write down each stage of a process in detail and agree to it, did the differences emerge. It required strong facilitation for individuals in the team to be honest about the way they felt about adopting what they perceived as 'someone else's rules'. This was particularly evident with the more junior members of the team who may have felt inhibited by their position in the heirachy.

It very quickly became apparent that it was not the Pathway structure that was the threat; it was the process of writing the Pathway that challenged the team and would ultimately determine the success or failure of the ICP itself.

The importance of careful planning and facilitation of the Pathway process was the first of many lessons learned. It is essential that every member of the multi-disciplinary team involved in any aspect of the care or process covered in a Pathway, is involved in the writing and agreeing of the Pathway. Ideally this means involving every individual, not just every discipline. Resistance within the team to any part of the Pathway will affect the practical use of the tool once written, the delivery of care to the client, and the success and efficacy of the Pathway itself. Even if a multi-disciplinary team appears to be working well together, when team members are asked to sit down together and to write and agree to each stage of a detailed Pathway of Care, it is surprising how many differences of opinion there are regarding best practice.

It took approximately two months to write the administrative Pathway and to gain agreement with both the administrative and clinical staff on its content. The process mapping exercise had brought together a disjointed, dysfunctioning group of individuals and over the two month period welded them into a unified, smoothly functioning team.

This does not mean there were no further problems. The effect of personalities within teams is a subject discussed regularly in corridors and between individuals, but it is a difficult and uncomfortable element of the team working equation to tackle openly. Personalities play one of the key roles in the success or failure of a project or service. It is for this reason that the process of writing Integrated Care Pathways, particularly in the multi-disciplinary, multi-agency environment characteristic of community and mental health services, cannot and must not be rushed. It takes time for individuals to reflect on and adjust to what will inevitably bring some changes to their working practice. If the process is to be a success, each individual must feel an active part of that change and must not be left with the feeling that the changes were imposed. It is often the most reluctant member of the team who will become the champion of the Pathway process if allowed the time and given the encouragement to become actively involved. Each individual will adapt at a different rate and, broadly speaking, the process must respond by adjusting to the slowest pace if it is to stand the test of time.

For any organisation to enable this process to happen, it is essential that a supportive culture is developed. To ensure effective team working there must be an environment for considering all ideas. Poor ideas frequently spark a train of thought leading to the emergence of a good idea, and if the culture of the organisation is one of openness and a willingness to listen to everyone's contribution, then good ideas combined with a willingness to explore new challenges will create an ideal environment for the introduction of Pathways.

Another mark of a good organisation is that it accepts mistakes will be made. By encouraging a culture of it being 'all right' to admit mistakes, it is possible for a team to understand these mistakes, to be creative and to take risks and suggest innovative changes. Such a culture leads to a proliferation of new ideas and changes to existing practice, and a good environment for the writing and development of working Pathways.

The administrative Pathway in Hounslow and Spelthorne was finally implemented in June 1992 and proved a tremendous success. Not only was the team then able to function supported by a clear, agreed protocol for each stage of the referral process, but the roles of individual members and their relationships with each other and the clinicians had been clarified. Figure 10.1 sets out the Administrative Pathway which became the first pilot ICP within the department of child and adolescent psychiatry.

The process of setting up a clinical Pathway

Following the success of the administrative ICP, morale soared and a decision was soon made to embark on the writing of a second Pathway. This time it was to be a clinical Pathway. At this time, the department of child and adolescent psychiatry had been successful in gaining project monies from a government funding initiative. Two highly skilled and experienced nurse practitioners and a secretary were recruited. The aim of the project was to develop a new and innovative model of working for the care of clients within a defined geographical area. The local area had high levels of deprivation with large numbers of families in council accommodation, on income

General pre-assessment (ICP:HA1) (pilot)

NAME (of child)	DATE	M	UM		DATE	M	UM
1 Receive phone call 2 Receive supporting letter and date stamp 3 Within one week: 3.1 Office manager identifies contract: 3.11 Existing contract ☐ 3.12 GPFH ☐ 3.13 ECR ☐ 3.2 Check whether known to the service in the past: 3.21 If family known, pull the file 3.3 Pass to consultant's secretary 3.31 Complete front sheet 3.32 Put in the consultant's tray for initial screening. 3.4 Process according to contract as follows: 3.41 For existing contract: Accept referral and enter in the computer registration. Allocate registration number and identify locality (same day). 3.42 For GPFH: Phone GPFH business manager to authorise the referral (same day). Accept referral and enter in the computer registration. Allocate registration number and identify locality (same day). 3.43 For ECR: Complete the 'Request for Authorisation' form and send to care group manager. Care group manager check form and fax/send to purchasers (within 2 working days) Care group manager receive authorisation from purchasers (within a week)				Care group manager inform office manager of the authorisation (same day). Accept referral and enter in the computer registration. Allocate registration number and identify locality (same day). 4 At allocations meeting: 4.1 Office manager brings referral to weekly allocations meeting (Tuesdays) 4.2 Send standard letter to parents requesting permission for reports. 4.3 Consultant screens for waiting list category: (a) Category One ☐ (b) Category Two ☐ (c) Category Three ☐ (d) Category Four ☐ 4.5 Send acknowledgement letter to GP (if not the referrer and if known) (same day as allocations meeting) 5 Once parents give consent, request information from the following (if requested by the consultant) and receive reply within two weeks: (a) School ☐ (b) Educational psychology ☐ (c) Educational welfare officer ☐ (d) Social services ☐ (e) Speech therapy ☐ (f) Occupational therapy ☐ (g) Physiotherapy ☐ (h) Health visitors ☐ (i) Specialist services ☐ (j) Other hospitals ☐ (k) Court welfare officers ☐ (l) Probation officers ☐ (m) Voluntary agencies ☐ (n) Medical notes ☐ (o) Other ☐			

Fig. 10.1   Pilot administrative ICP.

NAME (of child)	DATE	M	UM		DATE	M	UM
6 At allocation:				7.2 Copy letter goes to the referrer (and the GP if not the referrer) the same day as 7.1.			
6.1 Consultant allocated case to outpatient worker(s)							
6.2 Outpatient worker gives secretary the file with details of time/place/date/clinician for diagnostic appointment.				8 Secretary or outpatient worker enters the appointment in the office diary.			
7 Either:				9 Parents confirm appointment within time set on appointment letter.			
7.1 Secretary sends diagnostic appointment letter to (or phones) the patient's parents/ carer/social worker (if the child is in care) within 2 days.				10 Either:			
				10.1 Family unable to attend appointment – offer alternative appointment.			
or:				or:			
Outpatient worker phones the patient's parents/carer/social worker (if the child is in care) within 2 days.				10.2 Family fail to confirm: send standard letter to referrer and GP.			

Fig. 10.1 *continued.*

support, single parent families, families with over five children, high numbers of children on the At Risk Register and a large number of families without cars.

To evaluate the project it was necessary to document the new service developments in a way which allowed regular review, providing comprehensive information for audit. It was essential that the aims and outcomes of the new services were documented in a way which could be scrutinised and challenged.

Integrated Care Pathways were clearly ideal for this, and the clinical team set about writing a Pathway for the first of their new services: the brief intervention service for pre-school children with behavioural problems. The need to document the new service using a logical step-by-step approach served to help the team focus on the processes of care and ensure that each stage was fully thought through. The Pathway evolved, beginning with the setting of criteria for referral and progressing through the assessment, treatment, evaluation and finally the discharge stages.

When developing this first clinical Pathway, the team set out a general framework which would then be the template when writing any future community or mental health Pathways within Hounslow and Spelthorne:

- The Pathway must relate to a targeted group such as patients, clients, families or carers. This group may be defined in any appropriate way, for example by diagnostically related groups or a set of presenting problems or symptoms. It is often necessary to sub-categorise the target groups, for example by age band and severity or complexity.
- The Pathway must define the best clinical practice for that target group as agreed by those providing the care or input.
- The Pathway must be designed to fit the average, most typical case within that target group or be written to reflect the expected range.

Other optional components which are desirable, but not absolutely essential, when designing a community mental health Pathway include:

- Standards written into the Pathway
- Scales for the measurement of clinical effectiveness integrated into the Pathway
- Satisfaction questionnaires for the client, staff and referrer integrated into the Pathway
- Expected aims and anticipated outcomes for the Pathway
- Integrated records consisting of identified problems, goals, plans and notes with their own built-in variance analysis recording mechanism (Fig. 10.2)

In the case of the pilot, the clinical team chose to include the first of the three optional elements described above when writing the Pathway. For each appropriate task standards were agreed and written into the Pathway. The method of recording variances throughout the Pathway (see Chapter 3) meant that the new clinical service automatically had a built-in audit tool (Fig. 10.3).

Problems encountered along the way included the level of clinical detail that should go into the Pathway and the decision as to whether or not problem-orientated records should form part of the Pathway document. Problems of this nature were only resolved with discussion and careful thought about what the team would ultimately like to get out of the process. Once the team had carefully considered the benefits of Pathway use to their clinical research and evaluation, and the effect on preventing duplication of records, they were keen to include the integrated records with regular variance tracking.

Another issue was that of clinical judgement when using Pathways. Pathways of Care do not in any way compromise or interfere with the exercising of clinical judgement in individual cases. A Pathway sets out a protocol for the best agreed clinical practice for an identified target group, and then allows the clinician to focus on any variances that will be necessary

Problem and goal sheet

Problem no.	Problems	Date identified	Goal no.	Goals	Date to be achieved	Met (sign.)	Unmet (sign.)

Plan and notes sheet

Date of plan	Plan no.	Plan	Date to be achieved	Met (sign.)	Unmet (sign.)	Notes

Fig. 10.2 Format for the 'problem, goal, plan and notes' recording system.

to tailor the service to the particular individual in question and to retro-spectively audit the profile of service delivery for each client group.

Pathways do not limit clinicians to adherence to a set route, but ensure that important, agreed standards are met or at least monitored. They help to structure and focus individual clinicians and departments with regard to the modes of assessment and treatment that they offer; they support clinical supervision and contribute to audit and the training of new or less experienced staff.

Once a good Pathway is written it becomes an integral part of clinical practice and can be usefully added to the information shared with referrers, purchasers and also clients and carers themselves. This clear structure supports the mutual agreement of expectations, so often cited as the underlying cause of disagreements between individuals, departments and agencies.

The first clinical Pathway in Hounslow was an unqualified success, probably due to the subject area chosen, which lent itself readily to the Pathway process. Once again, the critical ingredient for the success of the Pathway was the involvement of all those with a role to play in the service delivery, in the construction of the Pathway document. The Pathway was owned by all members of the original clinical team throughout the process.

ICP PATHWAY – BRIEF INTERVENTION SERVICE PROJECT
Department of Child and Adolescent Psychiatry

Patient's ICP no . . . .

Screening – section criteria
(a) AGE   [   ]   YEARS   [   ]   MONTHS

(b) PRESENTING PROBLEMS
. . . .
. . . .
. . . .
. . . .

(c) MEDICAL AETIOLOGY?   [   ]

(d) DURATION OF PROBLEM   [Weeks   ]

(e) GP/HV/OTHER ADVICE SOUGHT?   [Y/N]

(f) IF YES, WHO? . . . .

	DATE TO BE ACHIEVED	DATE & INITIALS	
		MET/ YES	UNMET/ YES
1. Date referral received in department: ___ / ___ / ___			
2. Consultant selects for BIS Project within three working days.			
3. Behaviour nurse specialist confirms selection for BIS waiting list within two working days.			
4. Referral passed to: (a) BIS secretary if selected for BIS project (b) Consultant if rejected from BIS project			
5. Acknowledgement letter from consultant sent within two working days to: (a) GP (b) Referrer (c) Family			
6. Appointment letter sent to family.			
7. Waiting time [ ] weeks.			
8. (a) Attended 1st assessment appointment offered. (b) Attended 2nd assessment appointment offered. (c) Attended 3rd assessment appointment offered. (d) Discharged.			
9. At 1st assessment appointment: (a) Initial research evaluation completed (b) Assessment form completed			
10. Assessment summary completed within three working days of child's attendance.			
11. Final research evaluation completed following last attendance.			
12. If family discharged earlier than planned or if family do not attend: final research evaluation form sent to family for completion.			

Fig.10.3   Clinical ICP for brief intervention services.

It became very important that new members of staff joining the team were fully inducted into the philosophy and reasons for using Pathways as well as in the practical use of them. Without a clear understanding of their usefulness, the ICP could easily be treated as just another piece of excessive, time-wasting paperwork.

The members of the original clinical team had been newly recruited and were motivated and committed to a full and meaningful evaluation of their work. They were unfettered by historical service patterns and were establishing new clinical practices, providing an ideal environment for writing Pathways. The process was consequently less threatening and stressful than it might have been for those involved. The skills of the facilitator were tested throughout, ensuring that not only the loudest voice or the highest ranking team member decided the content of the Pathway; all views and opinions must be taken into account if everyone is ultimately going to have a commitment to using a Pathway and to making it an effective tool.

The main lessons learned from the pilot were the importance of selecting an appropriate target/client group for the Pathway, ensuring that there is a clinical 'champion', and having a committed facilitator ready to involve and encourage all members of the team and tackle any areas of resistance before the Pathway is sabotaged.

This chapter concentrates heavily on the process of writing the Pathway, rather than on the structure of the finished product, in order to stress the fundamental importance of this element of Pathway development, and to warn against rushing the process. If the Pathway is written in haste, the result is likely to be incomplete or poorly filled-in Pathway documents and resistance from uninvolved staff bent on undermining the success of the project. It is essential to take time and use a facilitator to lead the discussions, to ensure that all the key players accept the final Pathway content.

Implementing the Pathways

Following the piloting of the administrative Pathway, no changes were made to its structure for another two and a half years. During that time it continued to serve its purpose in monitoring the functioning of the general office and as a training tool for new staff.

However, following the piloting of the first clinical Pathway, several adjustments to its structure and content were made. The first alteration involved adding the integrated 'problem, goal, plan and notes' record to the existing Pathway structure. The layout of these combined records was designed to fit in with the existing patient notes. Variance recording was added to the 'goal and plan' sections (Fig. 10.2).

These changes eliminated duplication within the patient record whilst building an audit tool into the everyday notes. For the first time outcomes of care could be monitored regularly and accurately against those expected for each category of referral. This was an exciting development as it allowed for objective monitoring of both process and outcomes for the individual and the target group, enabling the team to drive and inform an 'evidence-based contracting' process (see Chapter 14).

The way forward

By the summer of 1994 the Hounslow department of child and adolescent psychiatry had successfully piloted both an administrative and a clinical ICP. Key clinical, administrative and management staff within the trust were all of the opinion that ICPs had an important place in the development, monitoring and evaluation of quality service provision. The department was now ready to write more ICPs. The team considered whether to concentrate on Pathways for new developments only, or to attempt a Pathway which strived to capture existing services.

The three consultant child and adolescent psychiatrists were consulted. They were asked the simple questions: 'For which conditions are clients routinely referred to the department?' and 'What services do you currently provide?'. The answers, however, were not as simple or straightforward. It quickly emerged that it would be a major project to define and agree common categories of referral for families who received our services and to define the service elements that made up the packages of care that we offered them (Chapter 14).

The following six months were a period of painful but gradual enlightenment. From setting out to determine the next area in which to write a community mental health ICP, we had stumbled upon the most fundamental issue of all. If you are to write a Pathway, it is imperative that you know exactly who you are writing it for, who will be following it and what its content should be.

Community services are frequently characterised by an individual 'package of care' tailored to meet the vastly differing needs of a wide range of individuals. It is fundamental to good community clinical practice that services are tailored in this way, using an eclectic approach. The model of 'fitting the patient to the available services' is undesirable. For this reason professionals offer a variety of complex packages of care made up of a wide range of individual elements of service provision. These packages of care are individually tailored to meet the needs of each client depending upon their particular mix of presenting symptoms or diagnosis, and incorporating their particular wishes.

It was a daunting task to begin identifying common packages of care and anticipated outcomes when the individual clients would have such a wide range of needs and therefore possible outcomes of treatment. The thought of determining a cost for each of these packages of care hardly bore contemplating, particularly in view of the already complex requirements of the NHS contracting process. Faced with these facts it was clearly time to make some radical decisions. There seemed to be three main options:

(1) Abandon the Pathway model in favour of some general standards which could be audited traditionally and embark on a team building programme
(2) Pick out some discreet services which were readily definable and write Pathways for them
(3) Re-profile all the work of the department to incorporate costed care packages using Pathways

The team finally settled on the third option: to attempt the development of a new concept of Pathways in costed care packages.

The series of tasks required for this process is set out in detail in Chapter 14, which illustrates the use of Pathways in evidence-based contracting. This chapter will therefore concentrate on the development of the structure and contents of the new Pathways developed as a result of this overall process.

The department analysed two main areas of activity in order to identify the Pathways that required writing:

(1) The 'Categories of Referral' commonly seen in the department, defined in terms of diagnostically related groups
(2) The various components of the service which could be offered, defined in terms of a menu of service elements for each category of referral

The department then went on to group a number of service elements together to describe the basic care package for each category of referral, i.e. the various services required to meet the needs of each category.

Pathways were written for each service element, incorporating standards, aims and anticipated outcomes, scales for the measurement of clinical effectiveness, and client, referrer and staff satisfaction questionnaires. The problem, goal, plan and notes recording system was integrated into the process, completing the cycle necessary to monitor processes and outcomes both for the individual client and with regard to the more general aspect of target groups of common categories of referral. Figures 10.4 and 10.5 illustrate the structure and content of the first drafts of these new comprehensive Pathways.

GENERAL PRE-ASSESSMENT (ICP:HA1)

Aim: To receive and screen a referral, process it through the correct contract and secure funding, seek further information regarding the referral, allocate to outpatient worker and arrange an assessment interview.

Pathway	DATE	MET (Initials)	UNMET (Initials)
1 Secretary receive referral phone call, and initiate ICP			
2 Office Assistant receives supporting letter and on the same day:			
2.1 Initiate ICP (if not already done)			
2.2 Date stamp letter			
2.3 Check whether family known to service in the past			
2.4 If family known, pull file			
2.5 Put file in office manager's tray			
3 Same day, office manager:			
3.1 Identify contract:			
(a) EHH Contract			
(b) EHH Contract/Hounslow Social Services SLA			
(c1) EHH Contract Satellite Clinic (please state)			
(c2) GPFH family in EHH Contract Satellite Clinic (please state)			
(d) GPFH/ECR Satellite Clinic (please state)			
(e) GPFH Block Contract (please state)			
(f) GPFH Cost per Case Contract (please state)			
(g) GPFH Cost per Case (please state)			
(h) ECR (please state)			
(i) Other (please state)			
3.2 Note family's name in office manager's diary			
3.3 Identify consultant responsibility:			
Dr X			
Dr Y			
Dr Z			
3.4 Allocate registration number:			
3.5 Record 3.1, 3.3 and 3.4 on database			
3.6 Put referral with ICP attached in consultant's tray			
4 Within one working day:			
4.1 Consultant screen referral and note waiting list category:			
Category 1			
Category 2			
Category 3			
Category 4			
Category 5			
Category 6			
Comments:			
4.2 Consultant tick boxes (see 8) to request further information			
4.3 Consultant put referral with ICP attached in office manager's tray			
5 Within five working days, office manager processes referral according to contract as follows:			
5.1 For EHH Contract, EHH Contract/Hounslow, Social Services SLA, EHH Contract Satellite Clinics, GPFH/ECT Satellite Clinics: Go to 6			
or			
5.2 For GPFH Block Contract, GPFH Cost per Case Contract, GPFH Cost per Case, or GPFH family in EHH Satellite Clinic:			
5.21 Phone GPFH business manager to authorise referral			

5.22 GPFH business manager either:
  a) give authorisation immediately
     or
  b) phone back and give authorisation within five working days			

GENERAL PRE-ASSESSMENT (ICP:HA1)

Pathway	DATE	MET (Initials)	UNMET (Initials)
5.23 Record outcome in GPFH contracts book			
or			
5.3 For ECR:			
5.31 Type out 'Request for Elective ECR Form' onto computer			
5.32 Phone ECR manager in appropriate health authority and inform him/her of the request for an elective ECR			
5.33 Follow phone call up with a faxed 'Request for Elective ECR' form within five working days:			
5.34 Receive authorisation from ECR manager to proceed with: Assessment Y N Treatment Y N Comments:			
5.35 Record outcome in ECR contracts book			
6 Office manager pass all information including ICP to consultant's secretary			
7 Within three working days, consultant's secretary:			
7.2 Complete front page sheet on database			
7.3 Send standard 'referrer acknowledgement' letter to: Referrer GP (if not the referrer)			
7.4 Send standard 'acknowledgement and permission to request reports' letter to parents			
8 Within two days of permission being given by parents, send standard letters to request fuller information from the following sources:			

	Consultant request for further information (date)	Permission given by parents (date)	Letter requesting information sent (date)	Information received from various sources (date)
8.1 School				
8.1 Educational psychology				
8.2 Educational welfare officer				
8.3 Social services				
8.4 Speech therapy				
8.5 Occupational therapy				
8.6 Physiotherapy				
8.7 Health visitors				
8.8 Court welfare officers				
8.9 Probation officers				
8.10 Specialist services (please state)				
8.11 Hospitals (please state)				
8.12 Voluntary agencies (please state)				
8.13 Medical notes				
8.14 Other (please state)				

9 Consultant allocate case to outpatient worker(s)

Keyworker: Name _____ Post _____
Other Worker: Name _____ Post _____
Other Worker: Name _____ Post _____

10 Within same day, outpatient worker complete 'pink allocation form' and put in office manager's tray

11 Same day as receiving 'pink allocation form', office manager record allocated outpatient workers on database.

12 Outpatient worker note on the ICP the date/time/venue/outpatient worker for the assessment interview to be offered

	Date	Time	Venue	Outpatient worker
Assessment interview offered				
Assessment interview offered				
Assessment interview offered				
Assessment interview offered				

Fig. 10.4 General pre-assessment ICP.

GENERAL PRE-ASSESSMENT (ICP:HA1)

Pathway	DATE	MET (Initials)	UNMET (Initials)

13 Either:
13.1.1 Outpatient worker phone family and offer assessment interview
13.1.2 Family confirm appointment over the phone:
 	
    Assessment interview confirmed for   [Date] [Time] [Venue] [Outpatient worker]
13.1.3 Outpatient worker enter assessment interview data on database
13.1.4 Outpatient worker enter into the appointment diary:
    a) assessment interview date, time and outpatient worker
    b) venue and room booked
13.1.5 Outpatient worker put notes with ICP attached in secretary's tray
13.1.6 Within two working days, secretary send standard 'offer letter' following telephone conversation to:
    Parents
    Copy to referrer
    Copy to GP (if not the referrer)
 	
    or
13.2.1 Secretary phone family and offer assessment interview
13.2.2 Family confirm appointment over the phone:
 	
    Assessment interview confirmed for   [Date] [Time] [Venue] [Outpatient worker]
13.2.3 Secretary enter assessment interview date on database.
13.2.4 Secretary enter into the appointment diary:
    a) assessment interview date, time, and outpatient worker
    b) venue and room booked
13.2.5 Within two working days, secretary send standard 'offer letter' following telephone conversation to:
    Parents
    Copy to referrer
    Copy to GP (if not the referrer)
 	
    or
13.3.1 Outpatient worker put notes with ICP attached in secretary's tray and inform secretary of assessment interview date, time, venue and room booked.
13.3.2 Outpatient worker enter assessment interview date on database.
13.3.3 Outpatient worker enter into the appointment diary:
    a) assessment interview date, time, and outpatient worker
    b) venue and room booked
13.3.4 Within two working days, secretary send standard 'offer letter', including:
    Date of confirmation of attendance [   ]
    to:
    Parents
    Copy to referrer
    Copy to GP (if not the referrer)
14 Either:
14.1 Family confirm appointment within time set out in 'offer letter'
    or:
14.2 Family unable to attend appointment – offer alternative appointment
    or:
14.3 Family fail to confirm:
    Offer second appointment.
    Offer third appointment.
15 If family fail to confirm three appointments discharge and send standard letter to:
    Parents
    Copy to referrer
    Copy to GP (if not the referrer)			

Anticipated outcome: Patient records containing all appropriate information available to be with allocated outpatient worker for assessment Interview

Achieved: Yes [   ]
              No [   ]

Comments:
_____
_____
_____

Fig. 10.4 *continued.*

ATTENTION DEFICIT HYPERKINETIC DISORDER (AD/HD) TREATMENT (ICP:HC7)

Aim: To provide a comprehensive treatment advice and training intervention for a child with AD/HD and their family.

Pathway	DATE	MET (Initials)	UNMET (Initials)
1 Family attend 2nd assessment interview and outpatient worker:			
1.1 Complete PACS			
1.2 Take family history			
1.3 Give handout on hyperactivity			
2 Family attend 3rd appointment and AD/HD team (clinical psychologist plus two outpatient workers, one behind screen and two with family):			
2.1 Give out attention training handout			
2.2 Give explanation of attention training			
2.3 Show video			
2.4 Give out homework and diary sheets to family			
2.5 Record homework tasks on ICP record sheet.			
3 At next four appointments, AD/HD team review homework tasks, set homework tasks for next appointment, and record on ICP record sheet:			
3.1 4th appointment			
3.2 5th appointment			
3.3 6th appointment			
3.4 7th appointment			
4 Family attend 8th appointment and AD/HD team (two outpatient workers):			
4.1 Review homework tasks.			
4.2 Set homework tasks for next appointment.			
and AH/HD team (clinical psychologist):			
4.3 Repeat psychometric assessment, videoed by the two outpatient workers who score observations.			
5 Following 8th appointment, outpatient worker. ask secretary to send out repeat BEHAR questionnaire to school.			
6 Secretary send out repeat BEHAR questionnaire to school and request return within 10 working days: Date			
7 Secretary receive BEHAR questionnaire back from school within 10 working days.			
8 Secretary put BEHAR questionnaire in outpatient worker's tray.			
9 At 9th appointment, AD/HD team (clinical psychologist and two outpatient workers):			
9.1 Review homework tasks			
9.2 Set homework for next appointment.			
9.3 Repeat Berkely activity questionnaire.			
9.4 Repeat PACS			
9.5 Repeat Berkely parent interview			
10 Following 9th appointment AD/HD team:			
10.1 Review diagnosis and treatment within AD/HD team.			
10.2 Discuss and feedback to consultant.			
10.3 Assess the need for the Ritalin treatment package (ICP:SE1)			
11 At 10th appointment, AD/HD team either:			
11.1 Review diagnosis and treatment with family.			
11.1 Discharge from AD/HD clinic with a maintenance programme.			
11.1 Handover family to outpatient worker team.			
or			
11.2 Review diagnosis and treatment with family.			
11.2 Begin the Ritalin treatment ICP (ICP:SE1)			

Anticipated outcome: The child and family have received a comprehensive treatment, advice and training intervention related to AD/HD and have either been discharged on a maintenance programme back to the outpatient team or referred on to the Ritalin treatment ICP:SE1

Achieved: Yes ☐ No ☐

Comments:

Fig. 10.5 ICP for attention deficit hyperkinetic disorder.

Results

Many lessons were learned from the development of Pathways in a community mental health setting. There will always be a number of different approaches to the delivery of any service element. It is often necessary to review the service as part of the process of writing a Pathway so that the final document is a statement of the 'agreed' best clinical practice for the average client.

This chapter has repeatedly stressed the importance of taking the time to plan and facilitate the process of writing and agreeing Pathways. Adequate training related to the theory and practice of Pathways is essential, and including the use of Pathways in all staff induction programmes and personal objectives is helpful in raising their profile. In this way, the organisation demonstrates its commitment to Pathways and ensures that every individual is aware of the function and place of Pathways within the clinical and administrative framework.

It is important to reassure clinicians that Pathways will not restrict clinical judgement, and to give regular feedback to all staff involved in the recording process. Clear, prompt actions resulting from any areas where variance tracking has demonstrated the need for quality improvements or practice changes, will ensure that clinicians remain committed to the use of Pathways.

Figure 10.6 illustrates the use of Pathways to co-ordinate the multi-disciplinary care approach. Use of Pathways in this way ensures that, whilst activity is recorded by all staff in the various multi-disciplinary teams, the information is collated with a patient-centred focus in line with agreed good practice. Pathways ensure that all tasks required to enable the client to receive the best agreed care in the best agreed timescales, are identified and explicit. They also allow standards to be set and monitored in an efficient way using variance analysis as a method of exception reporting. The information available from this process enables effective audit of service delivery and therefore enables effective continuous quality improvements to be made. The use of the integrated recording system prevents duplication of recording, whilst enabling the collection of detailed client-related information.

The library of Pathways, particularly when aggregated into care packages for each common category of referral, is invaluable as a marketing tool when used to share information about current and planned practice and high quality standards. It demonstrates a service's commitment to continuous monitoring and improving of quality. As discussed in Chapter 14, Pathways can also be used to drive the contracting process by providing evidence to support best clinical practice and to calculate the implications of changes in case-mix, skill-mix and resources.

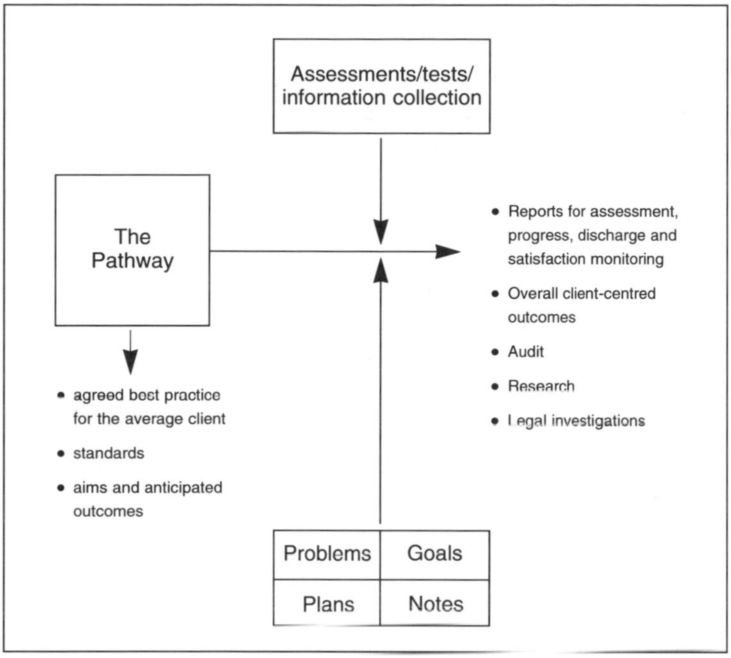
Assessments/tests/
information collection
The Pathway
• agreed best practice for the average client
• standards
• aims and anticipated outcomes
• Reports for assessment, progress, discharge and satisfaction monitoring
• Overall client-centred outcomes
• Audit
• Research
• Legal investigations
Problems
Goals
Plans
Notes

Fig. 10.6 The use of Pathways to co-ordinate the multi-disciplinary care approach.

The variance analyses from the first administrative Pathway piloted in the department of child and adolescent psychiatry raised a number of issues relating to inappropriate tasks being undertaken by particular grades of staff. This resulted in a full skill-mix review of the general office. This in turn led to the introduction of an office assistant post to deal with tasks such as photocopying, faxing and filing which had previously been undertaken by more senior members of the administrative team, and to the re-distribution of various tasks to streamline the administrative functions generally.

The same analysis also identified the long waiting time from referral to allocation of new cases to a consultant. The new care package model of working and information collection enabled the service to collect and break down the pool of referrals into the appropriate common categories of referral, and to plot the patterns of waiting times for particular groups as well as the rising trend in waiting times due to the increased rates of referral. Feedback to the purchasing agencies resulted directly in funding being given to address the problem.

Analyses of variance relating to the clinical Pathway in the department of child and adolescent psychiatry also raised some interesting issues which the service was able to tackle. One particular trend identified was that children referred with sleep disorders were attending the assessment and one or two follow-up sessions and then 'dropping out' of the service without completing the Pathway. This concerned the clinicians and a full investigation into the reasons for this premature, unplanned discharge was undertaken.

The results were unexpected. Rather than being dissatisfied, the parents were delighted with the behavioural programme and did not feel the need to attend after the second or third appointment. By learning from this experience, the clinicians were able to set goals which were better focused for that category of referral and were more realistic in terms of the number of planned sessions. Prior to the use of Pathways this trend had not been noticed. The effect on the service was to enable the tailoring of this service to meet the particular need by reducing the number of sessions and therefore the cost of that particular care package.

Another lesson which was learned was the need to plan regular 'analysis of variance clinics', which are built into the annual audit programme. Without this discipline it is easy to allow too much time to pass between analyses. In the same way that particular areas are chosen each year as warranting audit and evaluation, particular variances can be identified for detailed analysis.

Conclusion

It is essential for the long term success of the project that all members of the team are committed to the use of ICPs. Pathways will only ever be as effective as the least motivated person using them. For this reason it is worth giving serious thought and preparation to the process of writing the Pathways, their implementation and the ongoing support process. Including training on the use of ICPs as part of the formal induction process, and including ICPs in personal objectives will be necessary, if they are to be given ongoing commitment and are to be viewed as an important element of the care provided to the clients.

It has been learned from the experience of others that in most cases it is unwise to introduce too many Pathways at once. However, a common reason for their failure seems to have been the lack of involvement and therefore commitment by clinical staff using the Pathways, resulting in poor completion of the document. This is inevitable if Pathways are imposed by managers. Clinicians must drive the process and dictate realistic and achievable timescales if the process is to be a success. When introducing Pathways in any setting one of the main aims should be to design them in a way which integrates them with the recording system and makes them part of the routine of providing that care. Duplication of records should be avoided at all costs.

Practices which will support the success of Pathways include giving regular, appropriate feedback to all staff involved in using the Pathways. It is important that the findings quickly result in tangible and sensible action which clinical and administrative staff as well as managers can attribute directly to the use of the Pathways. Above all, there must be clinical reasons underpinning the introduction of Pathways if they are ever to be sanctioned and used effectively by clinicians.

Community mental health Integrated Care Pathways should be a clear, step-by-step description of the best possible practice for an average patient who is classified under a target group and appropriate subgroups. They should incorporate standards which ensure good practice and which are realistic, if not always achievable. If used to support evidence-based contracting, clear agreement should be reached between providers and purchasers as to the aims and objectives for doing this. Clinicians must always drive the process if it is to enhance patient care rather than just adding to the already heavy burden of administrative tasks.

The development of costed care packages supported by Pathways places services in a stronger position to respond to mounting competition created by the steady increase in GP fund holders and purchasing agency demands for evidence-based contracts. Whilst the model does not necessarily mean that services will be provided at lower prices, it does mean that purchasers will have the opportunity to study the outcomes of particular practices and that prices and contract activity will reflect the complexities of the care involved. This model will enable purchasers and providers to work together in the future to plan and develop purchaser and provider strategies which will meet the demand and which will be based on epidemiologically-related, needs-based assessments. The care package Integrated Care Pathways model can be promoted to purchasers as a way of supporting clinicians to improve the outcomes of their interventions and to enable the introduction of evidence-based contracting for the benefit of the population.

Perhaps in the future, community mental health Integrated Care Pathways could be re-named Anticipated Outcome Pathways?

Acknowledgements

Special thanks go to Dr Veira Bailey, Dr Caroline Hyde, and Dr Tim Hughes, all Consultant Child and Adolescent Psychiatrists at the Hounslow Department of Child and Adolescent Psychiatry; Dr Shanti Ponnappa, Consultant Child and Adolescent Psychiatrist at the Spelthorne Department of Child and Adolescent Psychiatry; Ms Alison Lyons, accountant; and to all who have assisted in the development of the 'costed care package' philosophy.

Further Reading

Light, D. & Bailey, V. (1992) *A Needs Based Purchasing Plan For Child Mental Health Services*. Paper published by Hounslow and Spelthorne Community and Mental Health NHS Trust, London.

'Costing for Contracting – The 1994/5 Contracting Round'; NHS Management Executive (NHSME) guidance FDL (93)59.

Chapter 11

Pathways for Stroke Care

Janet Brereton

Introduction

The use of an Integrated Care Pathway (ICP) on the stroke unit at Charing Cross Hospital, London, was achieved by the purchasers and providers of both primary and secondary care working together. The overall aim was to improve the quality of care for stroke patients and to provide information on that quality of care which could then act as a basis for local debate on stroke care services.

In the Health of the Nation document (DoH 1991), the Department of Health highlighted stroke:

> 'The term "stroke" encompasses pathological conditions such as cerebral infarction, intracerebral haemorrhage and subarachnoid haemorrhage. It is one of the commonest causes of death in adults. In 1989 there were 63 407 stroke deaths in England, approximately 12% of all deaths.'

In 1993 the local purchasing agency initiated a review of stroke services within the area west of London. To progress this work, they established borough-based stroke groups with a membership drawn from local acute and community providers, general practitioners, social services and the voluntary sector. The remit of these groups included:

- Reviewing and prioritising the recommendations from the purchaser's stroke review
- Debating and agreeing good practice guidelines and protocols in stroke prevention and care, including interface between the support agencies
- Agreeing outcome measures
- Debating and implementing an audit programme
- Evaluating and implementing change

In response to this review, Charing Cross Hospital decided to open a stroke unit to cater for patients within their catchment area who were suffering from a stroke. Following discussions with the purchasing authorities, it was felt that an ICP might provide the hospital with the means to:

- Assess whether standards and outcome measures were being achieved
- Look at the quality of care the stroke patients received
- Audit the service
- Implement and then evaluate change
- Act as a means of communication between different disciplines and services

The stroke unit opened in January 1995 and the Pathway was designed specifically for this unit, with the document coming on line at this time.

Developing the Pathway

The idea of developing a Pathway for the care of stroke patients originated during August 1994. The hospital and the community providers each had an ICP co-ordinator, and they facilitated the development of this Pathway. During the early stages the co-ordinators met with the lead consultant of the stroke unit, and they discussed at length the reasons for developing this Pathway and the potential benefits that might be gained from its use.

Further discussions then took place with members of the wider multi-disciplinary team, mostly on a one-to-one basis, so the co-ordinators could gauge the different opinions and views regarding the development of this Pathway. At this stage the various disciplines viewed the ICP as a method of co-ordinating, planning and evaluating aspects of care delivery for stroke patients. An overall positive response was received from all parties at this stage; the ICP was seen as a way of incorporating outcome measures directly into care, whilst also offering the opportunity to integrate the recommendations proposed by the borough-based stroke groups into clinical practice.

When initially embarking upon the development of the ICP, the aim was to set out what assessments, tests, referrals and treatments were required for stroke patients, and to obtain consensus on these issues between the different professionals. The team also set out to indicate who should perform each activity, and when was the most appropriate time for each activity. In this way the ICP would be able to encourage better co-ordination of all the inter-disciplinary processes of care delivery for the patients, so that care could be given in a timely manner.

The team also looked to the ICP to provide an audit tool, through the analysis of variances, that would allow the multi-disciplinary team to monitor failures or gaps in the continuity of care and correct them, whilst also identifying good practice.

Writing the stroke Pathway

'Ownership must lie with the clinicians and paramedical staff who have developed them (the Pathways); neither protocols imposed from the outside nor those dominated in their writing by one professional group are likely to be acceptable to staff not involved in their creation' (Heymann 1994).

With this in mind a meeting was convened for all key members of the multidisciplinary team who were at that time involved in the care and treatment of stroke patients. At this time the staff who would be working on the new stroke unit were not yet appointed and hence could not be part of the authoring team, although it would have been ideal to have developed the initial Pathway with the team that would eventually be using the ICP document day to day. The team included the occupational therapist, a ward sister, physiotherapist, consultant, head nurse, dietitian, speech and language therapist, social worker, pharmacist and a representative from the community team (Fig. 11.1).

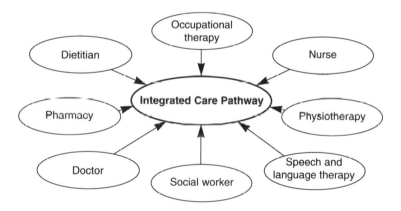

Fig. 11.1 Multi-disciplinary team involved in writing the stroke ICP.

Most of the team had previously been involved in the development of other ICPs within the acute hospital setting, which made it unnecessary to explain the use of a Pathway and its potential benefits to the team. However, it is very important to do this when writing a new Pathway with an inexperienced team.

Prior to the inaugural meeting, the hospital's ICP co-ordinator set out a basic draft of a stroke Pathway. This included suggestions for practice, based on research evidence and the recommendations from the borough-based stroke groups. This draft was sent out to all members of the authoring team, with an accompanying letter explaining that this draft was to act as a basis for discussion and to prompt ideas from all members of the team. The co-ordinator had found from previous experience that staff often find it easier to work from a suggested draft and to edit and criticise it, rather than start from a blank sheet of paper. Yet she was careful not to let the team feel that this draft was being imposed on them, but to ensure that local ownership of the developing Pathway was always held with the clinical team.

At the meeting all members of the team described the role each discipline plays in the care and treatment of the stroke patient, and through this the team built up understanding of each other's role. Fortunately the team had an open atmosphere from the start, with all members confident in expressing their opinions and contributions to care. The team must be aware that less can be achieved if the person with the loudest voice is allowed to dominate the discussions. The co-ordinator should be sensitive to this at all team meetings.

Due to the complexities of stroke care and treatment, and the wide range of abilities and conditions of the stroke patients, the team had to set boundaries within which the Pathway would function. For instance, who or which stroke patients should this Pathway be for? Should it be written for all stroke cases, or for the rehabilitation phase only, or for the first week of assessments only? The new stroke unit had definitive admission criteria for its patients, which delivered the opportunity to include all the unit's patients for this Pathway.

The source of admission for the unit's patients also posed a problem, as patients came from casualty, or via direct referrals from general practitioners in the community, or could be transferred from other wards within the hospital. Discussion focused on the difficulties of designing one Pathway for all the different sources of admission, and questioned whether a number of different Pathways could be written to accommodate the different sources of admission. This was deemed as too complicated for the first pilot Pathway, so the team decided to write one single stroke Pathway for all patients admitted to the stroke unit, from whatever source. If variances occurred, these would be recorded and reviewed after the pilot and the situation reconsidered.

The structure of the Pathway was another issue that needed to be addressed. The team decided that to start with, the Pathway would only cover the first week of admission and the last two weeks leading up to discharge. This was due mainly to the complexities of the condition, with the resulting variability between patients and their differing lengths of stay in hospital. The admission and discharge phases are the periods when care is at its most co-ordinated, and therefore easier to map out. The discharge phase is also a busy and complicated time, with the involvement of many disciplines and agencies from the acute and community settings; a Pathway

would enable the discharge preparations to be better managed and organised.

With these issues resolved, the team started to set out the content of each
day of the Pathway. Current practice, roles and activities of the various
disciplines were reviewed, so that duplication could be reduced and the gaps
in care plugged. A literature search, together with the recommendations of
the stroke groups, provided research-based evidence for aspects of care
included in the Pathway, which is important when setting out protocols for
clinical practice, as suggested by Wilder (1995): 'Protocols should be
consistent with any national recommended actions and take into account any
recent research'.

The ICP included outcome measures, standards of care and protocols of
recommended practice. For example, outcome measures were used on
particular days of the Pathway to provide the team with an indication of
whether the Pathway was appropriate and achieving good outcomes for the
patients. These outcome measures included the incidence of pressure sores,
deep vein thrombosis and contractures, and were assessed as part of the ICP
on specified days. The hospital had policies, which included the maintenance of certain standards of care, and the ICP included these standards,
so the Pathway could then act as a monitoring tool for standards; for
example, one standard was that all patients should receive a multi-
disciplinary assessment within two working days from admission. This
standard was set into the appropriate day on the ICP and then reviewed as to
whether it was or was not being achieved, through the analysis of variances
from the Pathway.

Protocols or guidelines for practice are available for all disciplines, yet it is
the integration of these protocols into clinical practice that can be difficult.
The team used guidelines for care from the Royal College of Physicians
(1994), and local pharmacy protocols for drug administration.

It took the multi-disciplinary team three meetings to discuss what should
be included in the ICP, and fortunately the meetings were well attended by
all staff. The consultant was able to attend all sessions, so many issues could
be sorted out during the developmental stages, such as drug protocols and
assessments, confirming comments by Riches *et al.* (1994) that 'the initial
meeting of all those involved can often iron out anomalies in care'. Poorly
attended meetings make the development and writing process much longer,
as difficult issues requiring discussion need the input of a number of disciplines. Also, the issue of ownership of the Pathway can become a problem
if decisions are made when many of the team are not present.

Changes were made to the initial draft of the Pathway, on the content,
wording and design of the document, before it was ready to be piloted. The
language of the Pathway must be clear and unambiguous (NHSME 1992),

Patient name: _____

Hospital no. _____

ICP: Stroke

	ADMISSION DATE: / DAY 1 DATE:	DAY 2 DATE:	DAY 3 DATE:	DAY 4 DATE:
Clinical assessment	**Doctor's assessment and clerking (Standard neurological proforma)** **Confirm diagnosis of stroke** **Eligibility for trials** Nursing assessment • Waterlow score • 6 hourly neurology observations	**Stroke team review before mobilisation** • 6 hourly neurological observations • Weight • Height No signs of pressure sores No signs of chest infection No signs of DVT	**Stroke team review** 12 hourly TPR + BP No signs of pressure sores No signs of chest infection No signs of DVT Bartel Score: _____ (Stroke co-ordinator)	**Stroke team review** 12 hourly TPR + BP No signs of pressure sores No signs of chest infection No signs of DVT
Occupational Therapist	Interview and assessment	Assessment Advice on positioning Wheelchair if appropriate	Assessment Secondary disabilities prevented	Treatment programme Initial assessment completed
Speech Therapist	Dysphagia assessment as per protocol	Dysphagia assessment Screen speech and language Alert doctor to dietetic referral (if appropriate)	Discuss speech therapy with patient and relatives Provide written advice leaflets	Speech and language management
Physio	Assessment as physio protocol Lifting and handling assessment Tone and movement Chest/respiratory Advice on positioning	Assessment/treatment	Assessment/treatment No signs of new contractures	Assessment/treatment If requested speak to relatives regarding mobility No signs of new contractures
Social worker	Initial assessment: contact area social services (if appropriate) Interview patient/relatives about social, psychosocial and practical environment		Social and psychosocial support for patients and relatives Information and advice as required Counselling (if appropriate)	Contact area social services (if appropriate)

Treatment/ medications	Measure and fit TEDs if hemiparetic If incontinent, refer to continence protocol **Review current medication and document dose and frequency (liaise with pharmacy if appropriate)** Contact pharmacy for liquid medications if dysphagic If paralysis: prescribe 5000 u heparin bd If signs of an infarct clinically: prescribe aspirin 300 mg od		**Consider treatment of raised BP**
Diet	Food/fluid chart Fluids/foods orally unless dysphagic (as per dysphagic assessment) If dysphagic: Consider nasogastric tube Liaise with dietitian	Food/fluid chart	Consider enteral feeding if dysphagic Food/fluid chart
IVIs	**IVI if dysphagic**	**IVI if dysphagic**	**Consider removing IVI**
Discharge plan		Review social situation with relatives Complete social aspect of nursing assessment fully Social needs checklist completed	Contact community stroke team
Referrals	**Dietitian (for therapeutic diets/ impaired nutrition)**	Social worker	**Dietitian (if unable to take oral diet)**
Teaching/ psychosocial social support	Information sheet to relatives	Stroke co-ordinator to talk to patient and relatives Patient/relatives have a stroke booklet	Discuss risk preventions with relatives and patient
Radiology/ other	**CT scan** **US (lacunar/ hemispheric)** CXR ECG		Cardiac echo (if appropriate)
Laboratory	**FBC and U & Es** **Blood sugar** ESR Bloods		

Fig. 11.2 Pilot ICP for stroke patients from Charing Cross Hospital.

| Patient name: _____ | | ICP: Stroke | |
| Hospital no: _____ | | | |

	DAY 5 DATE:	DAY 6 DATE:
Clinical assessment	**Stroke team review** • *12 hourly TPR + BP* *No signs of pressure sores* *No signs of chest infection* *No signs of DVT* • *Waterlow score* _____	**Stroke team review** • *Daily TPR + BP* • *Weight* _____ *No signs of pressure sores* *No signs of chest infection* *No signs of DVT*
Occupational therapist	Begin self-care activities Formal assessment written in medical notes	Begin discharge planning Begin OT programme as per OT evaluation
Speech therapist	Treatment/management programme	Treatment/management programme
Physio	Assessment/treatment programme No new contractures	Assessment/treatment programme No new contractures
Social worker	Employment/DSS allowances/ finance discussed Advice to patient/relatives about finance matters Housing access/accommodation discussed	Counselling with patient and relatives Does case need care management to be arranged Yes No (Tick one) If yes, refer to duty social worker in area social service office of patient's home address Patient/relatives aware of Stroke Association

BOLD type: Doctors to sign   *ITALIC type: Nurses to sign*

Fig. 11.2 *continued.*

Patient name: _____   ICP: Stroke

Hospital no: _____

	TWO WEEKS BEFORE DISCHARGE DATE:	ONE WEEK BEFORE DISCHARGE DATE:	DAY BEFORE DISCHARGE DATE:	DISCHARGE DATE:
Clinical assessment	**Stroke team review** **Consider discharge date** **Case management meeting completed** Weight ___ *No signs of pressure sores* *No signs of chest infection* *No signs of DVT*	**Stroke team review** **Confirm discharge date** **Case management meeting** Weight ___ *No signs of pressure sores* *No signs of chest infection* *No signs of DVT*	**Stroke team review** **Fit for discharge tomorrow** Weight ___ *No signs of pressure sores* *No signs of chest infection* *No signs of DVT* Bartel Score: (Stroke co-ordinator)	**Stroke team review** **Discharge** *No signs of pressure sores* *No signs of chest infection* *No signs of DVT*
Occupational therapist	Case management meeting Home visit with family, client, community OT and other relevant team members completed	Case management meeting Home programme reviewed	Information about community support provided Questions answered	Follow-up arranged (if appropriate) Discharge
Speech therapist	Case management meeting completed Aids ordered if required	Case management meeting Refer to chest/heart/stroke voluntary services	Advice given to relatives OPD arranged	Discharge
Physio	Case management meeting completed Home visit with OT (as for OT see above) Community physio contacted re: discharge	Case management meeting Advice to relative/carers	Self management programme Confirm discharge with community physio OPD/treatment review arranged Transport arranged for OPD	Discharge

				Patient/relative has:
Social worker	Care management meeting	Case management meeting		
	If to be care managed:	Ensure relatives aware of discharge arrangements		
	• Refer for case management			
	Check level of domiciliary services required	Independent services alerted for starting date (Link this through named care manager in area social services)		
	Inform domiciliary services re possible discharge			
	• Home help			
	• Meals on wheels			
	• Special diets			
Diet	If for home enteral feeding, inform dietician of discharge date	Contact dietician if dietetic follow up/service support needed, e.g.		
		• supplements for discharge		
		• advice for carers		
Discharge plan	*Tick one:*	**Ring GP regarding possible discharge**	**GP discharge letter written**	
	Discharge back to referring consultant	*Initiate self medication policy if appropriate*	**Prescribe TTAs in the morning**	• *TTAs*
	OR		*Relatives aware of discharge tomorrow*	• *Multidisciplinary discharge letter*
	Discharge back to referring hospital– ring hospital to arrange a bed	*Order transport*	*Obtain TTAs on ward (PM)*	
	OR	*Relatives alerted to discharge date (stroke nurse)*	*Check transport ordered*	• *Community nurse letter*
	Discharge home	*Community nurse contacted re discharge*	*Speak to community nurse re discharge*	• *Outpatients date*
	Refer to pharmacist for compliance aid and assessment	*Local community pharmacist contacted (pharmacist)*	*Write discharge letter to community nurse*	*Discharge letter sent to GP*
		Pharmacy talk to carer re: medication	*Stroke co-ordinator: discharge reports all together (multidisciplinary form)*	
			Outpatients arranged (if needed)	
Teaching/ information	*Stroke booklet to relatives and patients*	*Patient/relatives understand discharge arrangements (stroke co-ordinator)*	*Patient and relatives understand all the discharge plan arrangements*	

BOLD type: Doctors to sign   *ITALIC type: Nurses to sign*

Fig. 11.2 *continued.*

VARIANCE TRACKING SHEET

DATE	DAY NO.	TIME	VARIANCE AND REASON FOR IT	VARIANCE CODE	ACTION TAKEN	SIGNATURE

BOLD type: Doctors to sign   *ITALIC type: Nurses to sign*

Fig. 11.2   *continued.*

making the document easy to use and comprehensible for all. The final draft of the ICP was sent out to the community stroke team for review, as well as to the Stroke Association (Fig. 11.2).

Developing the stroke ICP was a lengthy process, taking some months, but the support and commitment to the Pathway approach from all the disciplines, and their regular attendance at the writing sessions, ensured that a Pathway was produced and piloted.

Implementing the stroke Pathway

The ICP started its pilot when the stroke unit opened in January 1995. Training was given to all the staff who were to be working on the unit. Since many of the unit's staff were newly appointed to the area, it was important that they were all included in the training. The training sessions covered the following:

- Reasons for using the ICP
- How to fill in the Pathway document
- How to write variances
- When patients should be taken off the ICP
- How the information for the Pathway will be used
- Time for questions

The hospital's ICP co-ordinator spent time explaining to the staff that the Pathway is simply an anticipated plan of care and as such is not cast in stone. 'The ultimate responsibility for whether to vary from the protocol or not remains, and must remain, with each professional' (Layton 1993). This is important, as the staff using the new Pathway have to be clear that it is their responsibility to decide if the ICP as a plan of care is appropriate for their patient, or whether they need to deviate from that plan. When the Pathway commenced, the co-ordinator spent time with staff on different shifts, so that any problems could be discussed, and to provide more training as required.

A poster explaining how to complete the ICP document was designed and displayed in a prominent position in the staff coffee room, where it could be accessed with ease and could be glanced at regularly. This was felt to be a better strategy than setting the instructions out in a booklet that might get mislaid or left on the shelf.

The unit also benefited from a local identified 'link person', who was to liaise with the ICP co-ordinator. The link person was invaluable in getting the Pathways completed, whilst maintaining the momentum and co-ordinating the patient care on the Pathways.

Reactions from the multi-disciplinary teams were positive, as the Pathway was seen as a means of co-ordinating care, enabling disciplines to see what each other are doing, whilst enabling the collection of audit data about the processes of care within the unit. Once a pilot of 13 cases was completed and the results of the analysis were fed back to the local team, discussions took place on how to progress care through consensus, and issues that were causing problems were openly debated and resolved. These feedback sessions also provided a useful support mechanism for the team.

Difficulties and how they were overcome

Some members of the original team who developed and wrote the ICP moved on to new posts, so that new staff taken on had to be trained in the use of a Pathway that they had not previously been involved with. This was sometimes difficult in that the new members of staff did not have the same degree of ownership as the previous teams, and some of them were suggesting that care practices should be done differently from those stated on the ICP. Training sessions and regular feedbacks to the teams served to maintain a sense of continued local ownership.

Occasionally members of staff who were not from the stroke unit were drafted in from other areas of the hospital for a short spell of duty, and they did not always complete the ICP. This was mainly due to the fact that they were not familiar with the documentation, and when the unit was very busy it was not easy to find the time to train these staff members on the Pathway method.

As the stroke ICP covered the admission and discharge periods of care, a Pathway was not completed until a patient was discharged, which could take up to four or six weeks (sometimes longer). This meant that analysis and feedback of the pilot Pathways was slow. However, the ICP co-ordinator ensured that staff were kept informed throughout about how the Pathways were running, and indicated when the end of the pilot phase was in sight. This was important to ensure that the staff felt there was a benefit from the extra work they were putting into the pilot project.

At this stage of the Pathway project, the ICP was not replacing any of the other traditional documentation. The ICP simply acted as an information tool prompting decisions, as well as being a tool for the audit of care. Ideally, the Pathway should replace at least some of the current documentation. However, with this stroke Pathway this was always going to be difficult. Some of the core activities surrounding admission and discharge are very similar for the majority of patients, yet the actual input of medical, nursing and paramedical activities differs for every patient. Hence at this point in the project, particularly for the assessment stages, it was decided that the ICP would not replace current paperwork.

One concern of the team when the Pathway was being written, was the recommencement of the ICP two weeks prior to discharge, for the discharge phase of the document. It is not always easy to predict a discharge date with accuracy two weeks ahead of discharge. However, the stroke unit's multi-disciplinary team had regular team meetings to discuss patient progress and plan discharges; these meetings provided the opportunity for the team to decide when a patient was ready for the two week phase of the Pathway leading to discharge. In the majority of cases, the ICP was recommenced for discharge appropriately.

'Protocols on paper are helpful, but fall far short of delivering care in a manageable way. Paper is inherently inflexible' (Heymann 1994). This proved to be the case with the stroke Pathway, as when major complications arose, it was extremely difficult to change the anticipated treatments indicated on the Pathway. It was necessary at times to take patients off the Pathway and put them back on the ICP when their condition allowed. This is to be expected with the early stages of development of a Pathway in such a variable setting and with such a non-specific condition.

Getting medical staff to sign the document was also a problem. Despite the unit being run by one consultant, other medical teams also cared for their own particular patients. Difficulties were encountered trying to get all the different medical staff to complete their part of the ICP. This is a training issue; with sufficient training, all staff would have been ready and able to fully complete the document. It was hard to train all medical staff within the department of medicine due to pressures of time and work-loads. Since the validity and reliability of variance recording and analysis depends upon the staff recording their actions, this is an area that needed addressing.

One suggestion for the future use of Pathways within the unit, was to have a 'named nurse' acting as a care manager, to ensure that all the actions on the Pathway were addressed by the appropriate multi-disciplinary staff member and completed on the document accordingly. As staff become more familiar and comfortable with the document on the unit, they will feel more confident in its use and be able to train new members of staff themselves, without relying on a co-ordinator.

The initial pilot ran from January to the end of April 1995 – almost four months. Thirteen patients were included in this pilot. Following analysis of the pilot Pathway the ICP was changed both in format and content. During this stage of revamping the document, the pilot Pathway continued to be used on the stroke unit so that when the new version of the stroke ICP was ready to be fully launched by July 1995, a total of 25 pilot Pathways had been completed. Therefore, the time from the start of the pilot to full implementation was seven months, with a total of 25 pilot cases being run and analysed.

Results

'Once implemented, protocols need to be kept under review and revised where appropriate' (Wilder 1995). Detailed analysis was performed on the Pathway following the pilot, and then every 20 cases following that. All the information from the ICPs was put onto a computer database. Information collated included what variances were recorded, what outcomes occurred and what standards were achieved. The content of the Pathway was also reviewed in terms of how often particular activities were not relevant for the stroke patients, to ensure that those activities included on the Pathway were utilised in the majority of cases on the revised document. In this way, a Pathway can be made appropriate to current common practice.

The number of times an action was not signed for on the ICP was also monitored as an indicator of the reliability and validity of the analysis of variance. The NHSE (1995) suggest that conscientious recording and auditing of Pathways helps identify good and poor practices.

Information was collated on particular issues including:

- Length of stay of patients on the stroke unit
- Age and sex distribution of sample
- Sources of access to the unit
- Contributing diagnoses and co-morbidities
- Destination on discharge from the unit
- Complications
- Outcomes measure scores (Waterlow Score, Barthel Index Scores, etc.)
- Reasons for delays in discharge
- Reasons for patients being taken off the ICP
- Clinical content of the Pathway and its appropriateness

Interfaces between the internal and external agencies were also examined in detail using the Pathway, with particular regard to the timeliness of referrals. Any problems highlighted were then discussed with the group as a whole. Outcome measures like the Waterlow Score for assessing risk of skin breakdown, the incidence of pressure sores, deep vein thromboses and contractures, together with functional scores like the Barthel Index, all provided information on the level of care delivered in terms of its success in providing good clinical outcomes for the patient. Collating this information on admission and discharge enabled the team to look at the progress of patients during their stay on the unit.

The analysis of delays in discharge and the reasons for such delays provide important information enabling action to be taken to eliminate those problems; this data is collated without further audit beyond the analysis of the ICP.

At the time of writing analysis has only been performed on the pilot project, so it cannot be estimated what improvements the use of the Pathway has made to the quality of care provided within the unit. However, informal feedback from the staff using the Pathway suggests that it acts as a useful prompt and reminder of the care that should be delivered each day; in particular, when certain referrals should be made. It reminds staff to inform relevant members of the team that a new patient is admitted, and to ensure that the required tests and assessments are performed. Discharge planning is started on the day of admission for each patient, and thereby planned ahead, making the discharge phase of the Pathway far smoother for the patient. Discharge co-ordination is important to ensure that all agencies are fully informed of the discharge at the optimum time, and prevents any cases 'slipping through the net'.

The process of developing the Pathway itself had benefits as a team-building exercise. Everyone had the opportunity to see how the other disciplines functioned, and where difficulties could be avoided in the delivery of patient care with co-ordinated and well organised provision. As indicated by Layton (1993) standards of care are often tucked away in a handbook, and not routinely incorporated into routine practice.

This was one of the aims of the ICP within the stroke unit: to incorporate such standards of care into the routine of care delivery and clinical practice. This was achieved by including standards within the content of the Pathway, and then using the documentation of variances and their eventual analysis to indicate where standards were or were not being met, and highlighting the reasons for standards not being achieved.

Certain improvements in the quality of the patient care were achieved even within the pilot phase of the Pathway, due to the review of care practices from the analysis of the Pathway and its variances. One issue highlighted in the analysis was that when a patient was admitted to the unit at a weekend, the referrals on to other disciplines were sometimes delayed. This has been addressed on the rewrite of the document, to enable referrals to be made on the day of admission and these referrals to be checked the following day.

As the stroke unit opened at the same time as the Pathway was commenced, it is not yet possible to ascertain if any cost savings have been made, due largely to a lack of baseline data from the unit. However, any changes in practice can be costed, and then the costs of care can be evaluated over time. In a similar way it is not yet possible to review lengths of stay and changes that may be made following the use of the ICP, as the unit is also new. Therefore lengths of stay will continuously be reviewed to see if they are getting shorter, and alongside this, complications and re-admission rates will be assessed for patients.

Conclusion

The Pathway provides an ideal multi-disciplinary tool to audit the process of care. It is easy to use. It involves all the multi-disciplinary team in the choice and collection of audit data. It incorporates issues required by the providers and purchasers of health care, and focuses on achieving the best care for the patient. It facilitates multi-disciplinary discussion on the processes of care delivery, through team feedback of analysis data, and this in turn facilitates changes in clinical practice.

The stroke unit at Charing Cross Hospital used an integrated approach in the development and implementation of a Pathway for stroke patients. The work is still in its infancy, with plenty of room for improvement, but the work has begun and has huge potential. The use of the Pathway has already been useful in team building, both between the different disciplines and also between the secondary and primary settings.

In attempting to sum up this chapter, the author can find no better comment than that of Heymann (1994):

'sitting down together to agree on a common approach does more than just get a protocol written. It encourages communication in general. If the protocol approach is multi-disciplinary, so much the better. It must be beneficial for different professional groups to talk to each other about each other's perspective on patient care'.

References

DoH (1991) *The Health of The Nation; a Consultative Document for Health in England*. HMSO, London.

Heymann, T. (1994) Clinical Protocols are Key to Quality Health Care Delivery. *International Journal of Health Care Quality Assurance*, 7(7) 14–17.

Layton, A. (1993) Planning individual care with protocols. *Nursing Standard*, 8(1) 32–4.

NHSE (1995) Progress with Patient Focused Care in the United Kingdom. Nuffield Institute for Health, University of Leeds.

NHSME (1992) *Step by Step Guide to Producing and Using Profiles of Care*. Silicone Bridge Research Limited, Leeds.

Riches, T., Stead, L. & Espie, C. (1994) Introducing anticipated recovery pathways: a teaching hospital experience. *International Journal of Health Care Quality Assurance*, 7(5) 21–4.

The Royal College of Physicians (1994) *Stroke Audit Package*. Chameleon Press Limited, England.

Wilder, G. (1995) The legal implications of clinical protocols. *Managing Risk*, January, p. 5. Published by Merrett Health Risk Management.

Part 4

The Issues

Chapter 12

Pathways of Care, Clinical Guidelines and the Law

John Tingle

Introduction

Pathways of Care, clinical guidelines and protocols are all rapidly gaining acceptance in the UK health care environment as essential quality and clinical risk management tools.

The Department of Health (DoH 1996) fully support the concept of clinical guidelines as a mechanism for improving the quality of patient services by promoting clinical effectiveness. Clinical staff are also becoming more aware of these and other tools as an increasing number of articles appear in the professional health care press. A momentum appears to have developed for their creation and implementation. However, their use is not without controversy. Some argue that the use of these tools will result in the standardisation of medicine, with clinicians essentially following 'medical cook books'. Clinicians, it is argued, will lose a good degree of their clinical autonomy. Others counter this argument by saying that these tools are 'guidelines and not tramlines'. Effective use can result in an improved quality of patient care and can reduce the increasing complaints and litigation levels in health care. This chapter will be concerned essentially with the legal issues surrounding the use of these tools, particularly with clinical guidelines.

Definitions

On reading the professional press, books and journals on the subject, it quickly becomes apparent that there appears to be no agreed use of terminology to describe the quality improvement and clinical risk management tools that are being used. The term 'guideline' is seen to be used synonymously with care protocol, care pathway, practice parameter, practice guideline and clinical guideline. Authors use a variety of terms interchangeably to describe what appears to be essentially the same thing. The Institute of Medicine (IoM 1990) in the United States have defined practice guidelines as 'systematically developed statements to assist practitioner and patient decisions about appropriate health care for specific clinical circumstances'.

Lohr (1995) elaborates on this definition; she says that:

'implicit in this statement are certain emphases: first, rigorous, science-based procedures for development; second, health care decision making that involves both clinicians and patients; third, a focus on specific clinical circumstances, including the full range of clinical conditions and problems with which primary care physicians deal, rather than simply individual technologies or specific procedures; and fourth, an assumption that guidelines will be practical, explicit working documents, not just lengthy compilations of the literature'.

This definition helps focus the creator of tools on an appropriate definition to adopt. It is, however, the ideas behind the concept that matter and not the label itself.

Throughout this chapter the term clinical guidelines will be used. The term is employed frequently in key UK literature, and by the Department of Health. The DoH (1996) employ a definition which is almost identical to that used by the Institute of Medicine (IoM 1990); that clinical guidelines are 'systematically developed statements which assist the individual clinician and patient in making decisions about appropriate healthcare for specific conditions'.

The growth and purposes of clinical guidelines

Clinical guidelines currently appear in the UK mainstream medical press at the rate of about one a week (Hutchinson 1995). In the USA the growth rate has been more over a period of about twenty years, with several thousand guideline-like statements and documents being produced (Lohr 1995). Clinical guidelines exist on a wide variety of matters. In the UK the Department of Health have listed some national clinical guidelines they commend and these appeared under cover of two DoH executive letters, EL(94) 74 and EL(95)115. They include:

• Management of asthma
• Management of diabetes in primary care
• Management of head injury

In the USA for example, the Agency for Health Care Policy and Research

(AHCPR) have published 15 clinical practice guidelines to date (Hudgings 1995) which include:

- Acute pain management for operative or medical procedures and trauma
- Urinary incontinence in adults
- Pressure ulcers in adults: prediction and prevention

A review of North American literature reveals that a variety of agendas exist for developers of clinical guidelines which do not appear to relate primarily to equality issues. Agendas generally also include helping to address medical malpractice problems and cost containment measures. Clinical guidelines can be seen to service a variety of masters (Lohr 1995; Klazinga 1995). The fact that clinical guidelines can have more than one central purpose raises some important legal issues which will be explored later in this chapter.

Locally produced, non-scientific based clinical guidelines: the norm

Centrally produced research-based guidelines are not the norm; most guidelines are locally produced and vary much in their quality. Lohr (1995) observes that most guidelines produced in the USA over the last twenty years do not measure up to basic criteria such as being science based, documented, unbiased, and clear. That same view can be taken of the UK, as Hurwitz (1995) argues:

'in reality, most published guidelines are not based on evidence, their recommendations being grounded, if at all, in consensus or individual opinion. Many are produced by groups without the expertise or resources to commission systematic literature reviews. In the case of general practice, recommendations may be based on false assumptions about the time and resources available for the care of one particular condition'.

It has been argued that the intended purpose of some guidelines is not always clear and that it is often difficult to determine the basis on which any recommendations are based (Hutchinson 1995; Cluzeau *et al.* 1995). This apparent variable quality of clinical guidelines raises an important legal issue if the clinical guidelines were to be used in court.

Evidence based medicine: do clinical guidelines actually work?

Evidence is scant on the issue of whether clinical guidelines generally can be said to work. Key questions in a court case may be: where is the evidence which supports your clinical guideline, and why did you use that particular clinical guideline in this case? Such questions raise directly the whole concept of evidence-based medicine. The scantiness of evidence in support of most clinical guidelines is worrying because it does affect the perceived credibility of the user from a lawyer and judge's viewpoint.

There is evidence that clinical guidelines can work. Grimshaw & Russell (1993) identified 59 published evaluations of clinical guidelines that met defined criteria for scientific rigour. All but four of these studies detected significant improvements in the process of care after the introduction of guidelines. The authors conclude that explicit guidelines do improve clinical practice when introduced in the context of rigorous evaluations. However, the size of the improvements in performance did vary considerably.

Bartlett (1995) also considers the question of whether practice guidelines work, and identifies a number of successful cases. The American Society of Anaesthesiology in 1989 approved standards for pre-anaesthesia care and intra-operative monitoring. As a result hypoxic injuries were reduced dramatically. At Harvard's nine teaching hospitals, the introduction of anaesthesia standards cut the average loss per anaesthetic by more than half between 1976 and 1987. These loss reductions allowed malpractice insurance premiums to be reduced. Bartlett quotes a study by Knox *et al.* (1994), which cites one carrier who promoted guidelines aimed at increasing use of baseline foetal monitoring, monitoring with pitocin usage, and other practice changes. As a result, changes in outcomes were observed before and after introduction of guidelines. The conclusion can be made that clinical guidelines can improve the quality of care and reduce liability risks for a number of conditions and specialities (Bartlett 1995).

The law

Some potential legal issues with clinical guidelines have been identified. These and others will now be discussed and examined more closely. The issues can be seen to fall broadly under the following headings:

(1) Legal discovery
(2) The legal consequences of not following a clinical guideline
(3) Clinical guidelines as evidence of the legal standard of care
(4) Negligently creating clinical guidelines
(5) Conflicting clinical guidelines
(6) Economically driven clinical guidelines
(7) Clinical guidelines as affirmative defences

Legal discovery

Clinical guidelines will be legally discoverable by a patient's lawyers in a negligence action because they could be relevant to the action. The creators of clinical guidelines should not fear this. The very fact that a trust or clinician develops and uses a clinical guideline shows that they have thought reflectively about the care environment and that they have addressed issues; this could go to their credit.

The legal consequences of not following a clinical guideline

Clinical guidelines are not 'cook books' and clinicians are expected to exercise discretion when treating a patient. Von Degenberg & Deighan (1995) state that guidelines do not preach 'cookbook medicine' but are there to support informed clinical practice and to encourage critical and objective analysis of current best practice. A clinician could be negligent if they applied a clinical guideline automatically without first assessing the patient. Clinical guidelines are not substitutes for professional judgement. There are too many variables in patient care for clinical guidelines to be applied automatically. Reflective practice is best practice. A clinician may decide that the patient's condition contra-indicates the application of a particular guideline and may decide to follow a different course. Alternatively a new treatment may be available and the clinician may decide to adopt the new practice. These courses of action would not be viewed as unreasonable by a court.

In determining clinical negligence the courts apply what is known as the Bolam Test. The court determines from medical or nursing experts in the appropriate clinical speciality what the ordinary skilled doctor or nurse in that speciality would have been expected to do in the circumstances of the case. In *Bolam* v. *Friern Hospital Management Committee* (1957) 2 ALL ER 118, the judge said:

> 'the test is the standard of the ordinary skilled man exercising and pro-fessing to have that special skill. A man need not possess the highest expert skill; it is well established law that it is sufficient if he exercises the ordinary skill of an ordinary competent man exercising that particular art'.

Did the clinician measure up to the standard of the competent practitioner by not applying the guideline and deciding some other course of action in the circumstances of the case? Some clinicians can of course do things differently to others but their actions must be supported by another responsible body of medical or nursing opinion to be proper.

The judge in Bolam further stated:

'I myself would prefer to put it this way, that (a doctor) is not guilty of negligence if he has acted in accordance with the practice accepted as proper by a responsible body of medical men skilled in that particular art … Putting it the other way around, a man is not negligent if he is acting in accordance with such a practice, merely because there is a body of opinion who would take a contrary view'.

Each case depends on its own facts. You cannot say that a clinician is automatically negligent because they do not follow a clinical guideline. They have a legally recognised discretion to exercise their own clinical judgement.

Clinical guidelines as evidence of the legal standard of care

There is a view that clinical guidelines are dangerous because they could be seen by a court to represent the legal standard of care owed by clinicians to patients in a particular case. Therefore if a clinician fails to follow a guideline, he or she could be viewed as being in automatic breach of their duty of care to the patient. This is not the case under the Bolam principle as long as the clinician's conduct is viewed as proper. Clinical guidelines are simply one of many sources of evidence about the standard of care in a particular case (Hurwitz 1995; Hirshfeld 1993). Clinicians can introduce legitimate clinical reasons why a clinical guideline was not followed. Variances should be noted and systematically analysed. The courts recognise that medicine is not an exact science. Feder (1994) puts this issue in perspective when he states:

'clinical and moral knowledge of individual patients is often subjective and implicit. This will remain the case, as will the intrinsic uncertainty of individual clinical decisions, no matter how many clinical trials are performed. These aspects of practice are not beyond research, but the methods are qualitative and do not fit the paradigm of "effectiveness" that generates clinical guidelines in their present form'.

Clinical guidelines should be seen as guides and not as prescriptive directions of clinical practice. However, as clinical guidelines feature more in cases, they will be an inevitable influence on lawyers and judges. The concept of evidence-based medicine holds that clinicians should practice research-based medicine. Reasonable practice, in the Bolam sense, then becomes 'best practice'. Possibly there could be a judicial drift or even switch from the Bolam principle as the concept of evidence-based medicine gains momentum. The Department of Health maintain that clinical practice is still insufficiently responsive to the changing evidence of best practice (DoH 1996).

Negligently creating clinical guidelines

It is possible that a guideline could be negligently drafted and when applied could result in injury to a patient. A key issue would be whether a reasonably competent trust or clinician would have adopted and used the clinical guideline. Other issues will be the design process and the criteria upon which the clinical guideline has been based. The guideline creation process should be fully documented. The steps taken by the health authority or trust to assess the suitability should be documented. The research methodology should be stated, as should the suitability and experience of design staff. It is very important to build a review date into the clinical guideline. New treatments and medical conditions arise and the skill mix that the clinical guideline was designed to operate with may have changed. You need to ask yourself, have you the resources now to execute the clinical guideline safely as you had when the guideline was created? Clinical guidelines which try to do too much could be viewed unreasonable; it is important to achieve a reasonable balance of expectations.

Bartlett (1995) offers nine strategies to reduce the liability exposure of guidelines, which include the following.

Scientific validity

He suggests that practice guidelines should be based on the latest scientific research, and updated every one to three years. Taking into account the observations quoted earlier of Lohr (1995) and Hurwitz (1995), that most guidelines are not science-based, this comment now assumes an added significance. The guideline maker may have to explain their guideline in court. As a matter of sound common sense they will no doubt have an easier task if they can prove that their guideline was based on scientific research and was reviewed regularly; such evidence would go towards establishing the reasonableness of the clinician or trust's conduct.

Treatment alternatives

When scientific research and expert opinion support different treatment approaches, these alternatives should be clearly indicated.

Patient preferences

Patient input should be elicited whenever treatment alternatives exist.

Deviations

The point is made that practice guidelines cannot anticipate every clinical circumstance, and that users should be encouraged to follow their own clinical judgement in exceptional cases. Clinicians should clearly document their reasons for not following the guideline. An example of what to say is: 'risk of procedure likely to outweigh benefits, in light of patient's condition'.

Conflicting clinical guidelines

Hutchinson (1995) stated that clinical guidelines currently appear in the UK mainstream medical press at the rate of about one a week. At that rate it is not beyond the realms of possibility that eventually you will have a situation where two organisations recommend conflicting advice. If a case ever went to court it might be the case of arguing whose guideline is better. The judge would not, however, choose between two responsible, though competing guidelines; both would be acceptable.

In the US, the situation of conflicting guidelines has occurred with mammography screening for breast cancer (Stason 1991). The American Cancer Society developed a screening guideline that recommended mammography every one to two years for all women 40 to 49 years of age, and annually for those between 50 and 74 years. The American College of Physicians recommended targeting screening in younger women, specifically those who are at a higher risk of developing breast cancer.

> 'Which guidelines should patients and providers act upon? The need is not so much to force uniformity among guidelines; uncertainties created by inadequate data are a fact of life and may allow multiple valid interpretations. The need, therefore, is at least to explain the reasons for differences clearly so that users can make informed decisions'. (Stason 1991).

The key point is to explain the reasons for the differences if there are any. This raises the question of who is to do the explaining. Clinical guideline developers should guard against rushing out material without an adequate survey of the word literature (Von Degenberg & Deighan 1995).

Economically driven clinical guidelines

A clinical guideline can be designed primarily to improve the quality of patient care. An ancillary benefit may be that the clinical treatment becomes more cost effective through efficiency; a matter to consider is when the clinical guideline is designed primarily to impose a cost reduction regime.

There is a danger that patient care and safety may be unreasonably compromised by clinicians disregarding good medical judgement in order to follow cost containment measures.

The courts recognise that trusts and health authorities have to work within limited budgets and that tough decisions have to be made on how finite health resources are distributed. A clinical guideline which is designed to make better use of scarce resources is commendable, but not at the risk of endangering the patient; a balance must be struck. Sir Thomas Bingham (Master of the Rolls) in *R.* v. *Cambridge HA ex p B* (1995) 2 All ER 129 stated the court's philosophy on the issue of NHS resources:

> 'It is common knowledge that health authorities of all kinds are constantly pressed to make ends meet. They cannot pay their nurses as much as they would like; they cannot provide all the treatments they would like; they cannot purchase all the extremely expensive equipment they would like; they cannot carry out all the research they would like; they cannot build all the hospitals and specialist units they would like. Difficult and agonising judgments have to be made as to how a limited budget is best allocated to the maximum number of patients. That is not a judgment which the court can make'.

The courts do not wish to become the arbiters of hospital waiting lists or to determine who receives treatment. If a health authority distributes resources in a way in which other health authorities would have distributed them, then broadly speaking its decision could not be challenged (Tingle 1993). Clinical guidelines can reflect economic factors but only in a reasonable way.

The dangers of economic driven clinical guidelines can be seen in the USA case of *Wickline* v. *State of California* (1986) Cal App 2d, 228 Cal Rptr 661. The California Medicaid program (Medi-Cal) refused a doctor's request for additional days of patient monitoring on the basis that they were not required under the clinical algorithms developed by Medi-Cal. The patient was discharged and subsequently developed complications. Cost-containment reasons had overridden the doctor's better judgement. The patient sued Medi-Cal for medical negligence in requiring the doctor to discharge the patient against the doctor's better judgement for cost-containment reasons. The court warned that doctors would be liable where they disregard good medical judgement by following cost containment guidelines when the outcome may adversely affect the patient.

The implementors of the clinical guidelines could also be liable in certain circumstances (Merz 1993). Segar (1995) has also argued that care paths must be scientifically based and never distorted solely to effect cost control or other non scientific support. The DoH (1996) takes a positive quality improvement view of the mission of clinical guidelines: 'guidelines are produced for the benefit of clinicians and their patients and are a mechanism for improving the quality of services, not for cutting expenditure'.

Clinical guidelines as affirmative defences

It was stated earlier that clinical guideline development is in its infancy in the UK and that British lawyers are just beginning to get to grips with the concept. However, in the USA where the clinical guideline concept has had about twenty more years to develop, some states have taken the concept to what can be regarded as the ultimate legal extreme, by using clinical guidelines as affirmative defences in legal actions. The state of Maine has led this development with its project, The Maine Medical Liability Demonstration Project (Smith 1993).

In Maine, to encourage doctors to practice less defensively, immunity is granted in the state legislation to those who follow certain practice guidelines. If it is uncontested that a doctor adhered to the appropriate clinical guideline, any suit against that doctor can be dismissed before trial. This strategy can only be employed by the defence 'as a shield and not by the plaintiff as a sword'. Projects are also being considered in Florida, Kentucky, Maryland, Minnesota, New York and Vermont (Bartlett 1995). Three years on from the initiation of the Maine project in 1992, not a single lawsuit covered by the clinical guidelines in the project has been initiated. 'Early experience suggests that plaintiff attorneys are reluctant to file a lawsuit if they do not expect to prevail' (Bartlett 1995).

Such projects would not find a place in the present English medico-legal environment where clinical guidelines are still in their infancy and such issues as defensive medicine do not pervade the tort reform agenda as much as they do in the USA.

Conclusion

Clinical guidelines are here to stay in their many manifestations. Nobody really knows whether they generally work but the conventional wisdom and the limited research says that they do. The key is to base them on sound evidence. The DoH (1996) has classified the types of evidence used in the guidelines. Those clinical guidelines which do not fall into one of the three stated categories will not be commended by the NHS Executive. Clinical guidelines should have a firm scientific evidence base. The developers of clinical guidelines should fully document the whole development process and should not be afraid to review them regularly. The key legal watchword is 'reasonableness'.

Evidence-based medicine and the DoH initiatives have started a momentum for clinical guideline development which will continue to grow. As clinical guidelines develop they will form part of the evidence in a court case and could be used for either inculpatory or exculpatory purposes (Hyams *et al.* 1995).

Lawyers and judges will inevitably get to know them and therefore they do maintain important legal implications. The benefits of having clinical guidelines seem, on review of literature in the USA and the UK, to outweigh the disadvantages. Reflective practice is good practice and clinical guidelines show at the very least that there is a controlled and reflective environment of care in operation.

Clinical guidelines that are developed solely for cost containment considerations are a double edged sword and it is pleasing to see that the Department of Health see clinical guidelines as an essential care quality improvement tool.

Clinical guidelines do not remove the clinical autonomy of the user and their legal accountability; this fact should be stressed in writing on all guidelines.

On balance clinical guidelines do *not* seem to expose the producer or user to a greater risk of liability than that which presently exists.

References

Bartlett, E.E. (1995) *Practice Guidelines: How Risk Managers Can Tap the Benefits, Avoid the Pitfalls.* Executive Briefing, Edward Bartlett Associates, Rockville, MD, USA.

Cluzeau, F., Littlejohn, P., Grimshaw, J. & Feder, G. (1995) Draft appraisal instrument for clinical guidelines. In *The Development and Implementation of Clinical Guidelines; a Report from General Practice* No 26, April. London. The Royal College of General Practitioners.

DoH (1996) *Promoting Clinical Effectiveness; a Framework for Action In and Through the NHS.* Department of Health, London.

Feder, G. (1994) Clinical guidelines in 1994. *British Medical Journal*, December, **309**, 1457–8.

Grimshaw, J.M. & Russell, I.T. (1993) Effect of clinical guidelines; a systematic review of rigorous evaluations. *The Lancet*, **342**, 1317–22.

Hirshfeld, E. (1993) Use of practice parameters as standards of care and in health care reform; a view from the American Association. *Journal on Quality Improvement*, **19**(8) 322–34.

Hudgings, C. (1995) Guideline development and dissemination programme; agency for health care policy and research, USA. In *Clinical Effectiveness from Guidelines to Cost-Effective Practice*, (eds M. Deighan & S. Hitch) Earlybrave, Essex.

Hurwitz, B. (1995) Guideline effectiveness; the pitfalls and obstacles. In *The Development and Implementation of Clinical Guidelines; a Report from General Practice*, no. 26, April. The Royal College of General Practitioners, London.

Hutchinson, A. (1995) Improving the quality of healthcare; the place of clinical guidelines. In *The Development and Implementation of Clinical Guidelines; a Report from General Practice*, no. 26, April. The Royal College of General Practitioners, London.

Hyams, A., Brandenburg, J.A., Lipsitz, S.R., Shapiro, D.W. & Brennan, T.A. (1995) Practice guidelines and malpractice litigation; a two way street. *Annals of Internal Medicine*, **122** (6) 450–55.

Institute of Medicine (1990) *Clinical Practice Guidelines; Directions for a New Program*, (eds M.J. Field & K.N. Lohr). National Academy Press, Washington DC.

Klazinga, N. (1995) Clinical guidelines bridging evidence based medicine and health service reform; a European perspective. In *Clinical Effectiveness from Guidelines to Cost-Effective Practice*, (eds M. Deighan & S. Hitch). Earlybrave, Essex.

Knox, G.E. *et al.* (1994) Obstetrical clinical risk modification; are medical malpractice lawsuits inevitable?. *Forum* **5**, 6–8.

Lohr, K.N. (1995) Guidelines for clinical practice; what they are and why they count. *The Journal of Law, Medicine and Ethics*, **23**(1) 49–56.

Merz, S.M. (1993) Clinical practice guidelines; policy issues and legal implications. *Journal on Quality Improvement*, **19**(8) 306–12.

Segar, G. (1995) Medical care paths can provide liability protection. *Advisory*, **XI**(3) 4–5, MMI Companies Inc.

Smith, G.H. (1993) A case study in progress; practice guidelines and the affirmative defence in Maine. *Journal on Quality Improvement*, **19**(8) 355–62.

Stason, W.B. (1991) Implementation of practice guidelines: the next frontier. *The Internist*, October, 9–12.

Tingle, J.H. (1993) The allocation of healthcare resources in the National Health Service in England; professional and legal issues. *Annals of Health Law*, **2**, 195–213.

Von Degenberg, K. & Deighan, M. (1995) Guideline development; a model of multi-professional collaboration. In *Clinical Effectiveness from Guidelines to Cost-Effective Practice*, (eds M. Deighan & S. Hitch). Earlybrave, Essex.

Further reading

For a contemporary discussion of evidence based medicine:

Cluzeau, F., Littlejohn, P., Grimshaw, J. & Feder, G. (1995) 'Draft appraisal instrument for clinical guidelines. In *The Development and Implementation of Clinical Guidelines*, Report from General Practice, no. 26, April. The Royal College of General Practitioners, London.

On the success of clinical risk modification programmes and clinical guidelines generally:

MMI Companies Inc. (1993) *Clinical Risk Modification; An 8 Year Data summary.* MMI Companies Inc., Deerfield, Illinois, USA.

For a discussion of a UK case on guidelines, procedures to follow when there has been an unsuccessful intubation:

Early v. *Newham Authority* (1994) 5 Med LR 214, discussed by Hurwitz, B. (1995): Protocols, guidelines and the law of negligence, *Clinical Risk*, 1(4) 142–6.

Chapter 13

Pathways of Care – A Tool for Minimising Risk

Jo Wilson

Introduction

Managing health care effectively depends significantly upon close monitoring of patient and family needs throughout the continuum of care. The more efficiently this is done, the more a provider unit's resources and management of risk can be promptly integrated into a flow of interventions which benefit patients; hence the high level of interest in tools like Pathways of Care. Purchasers are also interested in the tool as Pathways help towards a greater understanding of clinical processes, including clinical audit and risk management (Swage & Wilson 1995). Integrated Care Management views the multi-disciplinary approaches to collaborating care delivery by activity, cost and quality, using a process approach to problem and outcome based care delivery. Involving patients and their carers in determining the processes and outcomes of care provides a route to better communication, staff and patient satisfaction and overall improved quality of care.

This chapter deals with the use of Pathways of Care as a tool for minimising risk, looking at the risk issues inherent in managing the multi-disciplinary team in writing and using Pathways. There will be many questions posed which individual health care organisations must answer for themselves and relate to their own organisational culture and change management within their own Pathway project.

The definition being used for 'risk' is the potential for an unwanted outcome. This is as broad as a patient waiting too long in the outpatients department to a patient having the wrong operation or incorrect leg amputated, or even death. The quality approach incorporated within this chapter is that of Deming (1982): 'quality of care is getting it right first time and every time'.

Risk management is about the prevention of unwanted outcomes, involving the clinical team in minimising clinical risk, and avoiding negligence. It is the systematic identification, assessment and reduction of risks to patients and staff through:

- Providing appropriate, effective and efficient levels of patient care
- Preventing and avoiding untoward incidents and events
- Providing for comprehensive, objective, consistent and accurate communication and documentation of care

Pathways of Care represent a process approach to managing integrated clinical care. A Pathway is a staged plan that notes the appropriate use and timing of procedures in relation to patient recovery. The inter-disciplinary approach helps to reduce variation in clinical practices across the different care settings, whilst continuing to maintain quality patient care and enhancing clinical risk management. A variance from the Pathway is a deviation or detour from the plan of care and these are to be expected. Individualised patient care must allow for appropriate variations from the plan with explanations of the reasons for omissions and commissions in care. Variations from the Pathway are immediately recorded and acted upon through the care management audit problem solving process. These tools enquire into clinical practice and identify remedial factors to improve practice. Analysis of variance provides the 'window of opportunity' to indicate if things are missed or changed for specific patients, thereby demonstrating individualised patient care and reasons for omissions and commissions (Wilson 1992). Variance recording therefore acts as a communication tool where the patient is informed and part of the care process, and hence less exposed to unwanted outcomes or the need to complain about services.

Recently there has been an explosion of interest in Pathways and guidelines, reflected in a vivid debate ranging from 'the best thing since sliced bread' to cries of 'cookbook medicine' and fears of constraints on clinical freedom (Thomson *et al.* 1995). Pathways do not represent 'cookbook medicine' but are a truly integrated care management approach. Each Pathway is debated and agreed by a multi-disciplinary team to establish consistent and realistic goals and risk exposures. The team provides agreed guidelines which become a combined working document of patient care.

Clinical effectiveness

Clinical effectiveness as described in EL(93)115 (DoH 1993) clearly outlines the need for the multi-disciplinary team to identify and develop evidence based clinical guidelines or protocols of care. An integrated care management system focuses on the continuity of care by examining the organisation and management of care, and facilitating the smooth transition between hospital and home. This helps clinicians and managers to communicate the process, thereby managing and reducing clinical risk.

Integrating and designing the services around the specific needs of the patient promotes seamless care and aids the following:

- Reduces patient uncertainty and delays, making them partners in care with heightened public awareness
- Eliminates duplication and unexplained variations in clinical practice between the multi-disciplinary team members
- Improves resource utilisation and enhances efficiency savings, by incorporating medical advances, the increasingly complex decision making processes and a more explicit debate about the use of limited resources
- Improves patient care management and enhances family centred care and their participation in decision making
- Enables inter-disciplinary audit through goal setting, outcome monitoring and variance tracking, thereby improving the quality of patient care

Pathways provide a framework giving greater quality assurance, promoting timely, uniform quality and multi-disciplinary standards, with a focus on continually learning from and improving upon the process of care delivery. They help NHS trusts in their quest for continuous quality improvement, and minimise risk exposure by seeking better understanding and control of the care delivery process, to achieve cost effective accountability and to promote recruitment and retention of staff.

Pathways are part of an overall approach to proactive collaborative care, aimed at both improving quality and reducing costs, whilst modifying clinical risk exposure. They list patients' problems, expected outcomes, tasks or interventions within specific time frames required to meet those outcomes. Contingency plans can then be drawn up if the care differs from the plan. The multi-disciplinary team agrees the diagnosis to be used and then plans in a systematic way the guide or plan of treatment for each patient group. The care management system provides a set of tools to carefully manage the process, thereby optimising its outputs both clinically and financially, whilst also reducing the risk exposure.

Pathways differ from other approaches

The Pathway becomes the patient's case notes, a working document which has contributions from the whole multi-disciplinary team. The patient's history, assessments and physical examinations can become part of the Pathway. Everyone is then working from the same plan of care and the patient and relatives are partners in the care process, thereby improving the two main areas of risk exposure:

(1) Effective communication
(2) Appropriate documentation

Pathways offer a multi-disciplinary approach for describing appropriate evidence-based care, helping patients and professionals make decisions about healthcare and reducing variations in the care process. Variances are recorded and monitored, leaving room for justifiable variations in practice and plenty of scope for individualised care. Analysis of variances gives data about individual clinical practice and its supporting systems, enabling clinicians to make considered decisions about clinical practice.

Pathways provide an information basis for clinical and organisational audit focusing on specific circumstances, while taking account of organisational factors, community characteristics and other influences on health care delivery. Pathways also provide information useful for skill mix analysis. Based on data changes and costs, utilisation and health status outcomes relative to the implementation of Pathways can be measured and risk exposure reduced by better communication and documentation.

Health care risk management

Consistency of practice is important in all health care settings, to avoid conflicts and counterproductive processes. Pathways improve communication and the documentation of patient care. Currently care is recorded in various professional records up to eight times, with communication being haphazard and inefficient. Thus there is a need for an accurate and concise plan of care and a communication strategy. Pathways provide this interdisciplinary record and communication tool, promoting a collaborative care network which can start at the point of diagnosis, through any kind of health care setting, ending back in the patient's home when the total episode of care is complete.

In the professional liability arena, standards of care issues span across the health care network. Dual standards (when care is provided to different standards in the same trust, between different professionals) may produce a threat of exposure to the network overall. Many clinical negligence cases have used a dual standard of care within the same trust as an argument for plaintiff verdicts. Variances in standards of care and clinical practice within the same organisation can create liability exposure for the NHS trust or health care organisation.

There is also the question of appropriateness of care. Information to date has shown that concentrating on quality alone is not enough; as quality of care increases, the appropriateness of care decreases, resulting in unnecessary activities and increased costs. Pathways can help to address these issues by appropriateness of care, efficiency and effectiveness (Fig. 13.1).

Appropriateness of care
Pathways define the practice parameters addressing whether interventions should be done and how well, based upon research-based practice.

Efficiency
This is determined by discussing and agreeing how and when to undertake the interventions, and does it pay?

Effectiveness
This may be determined by examining the outcomes of care and looking at whether a particular intervention or activity worked, and whether it was worth doing.

Fig. 13.1 Appropriateness of care, efficiency and effectiveness.

Pathways decrease variability in outcomes, provide reproducible results and contribute to the development of quality assurance programmes, providing benchmarks for clinical audit and risk modification guidelines. They help to provide a controlled environment of care with everyone 'singing from the same songsheet' and thereby decreasing the frequency and severity of complaints and possible clinical negligence claims.

Quality assurance

From a quality viewpoint Pathways follow the quality cycle and feedback loop by describing what the health care team do, ironing out variability and risk exposure. Quality assurance is enhanced by ensuring the cycle is completed. Resource management is also facilitated by the completion of the cycle in the most efficient manner (Fig. 13.2).

The quality feedback cycle can be translated into the care management process of the Pathway cycle. Following the cycle can help with continuous quality improvements with benefits to patients, staff and the healthcare organisation. Cycles decrease variability in clinical outcomes and provide reproducible results which can tighten up the Pathway process and thereby reduce risk exposure.

Pathways can assist with the contracting and costing process by demonstrating quality, standards, inbuilt audit, outcome measurement and

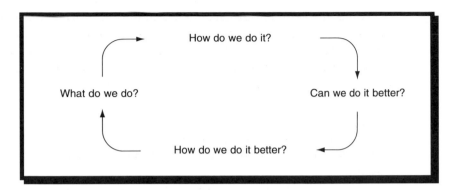

Fig. 13.2 Quality cycle.

clinical benchmarking, and with the information and activity data provided, accurate packages of care may be costed for both purchasers and providers of healthcare.

The second element of risk management to be addressed is in the project management of the Pathway system: how Pathways are initiated and then maintained as part of the health care routine.

Risk management

Risk management in this case is about careful planning to identify many of the risks inherent in initiating a Pathways of Care project and in the ongoing usage of the Pathways developed, and taking action to eliminate or minimise the impact of such risks. Understanding that risks exist is the most crucial step in the risk management process.

Risks to the best managed projects are inevitable due to the following often unexpected reasons:

- Number of people and disciplines involved
- Individuals behaving differently from the way anticipated
- Individuals over committing themselves
- Individuals' attention being diverted to more pressing issues
- Individuals not appreciating their role, which has not been clearly defined
- Under-estimation of education and training needs
- Unforeseen technical difficulties causing delays and despondency
- Unrealistic timescales are set
- External effects
- Losing impetus through poor project management, poor ongoing

education and support to staff, and insufficient induction of new and transient staff

Assessment and identification of risks will help identify the advantages, limitations and resource constraints in implementing a Pathway project and its ongoing support.

It is useful to identify the following:

- Insufficient, inadequate, obsolete or counterproductive procedures
- Problems with communication between different levels of work, the multi-disciplinary team, the interface between primary and secondary care and the external environment
- The criteria needed to support the data elements for obtaining quantitative and qualitative information
- The process and outcome criteria linked to the processes within the Pathways and their overall outcomes
- A lack of critical review of untoward events or poor outcomes, and an analysis of the strengths and weaknesses of the response

There are certain key questions which all organisations involved in Pathways of Care need to address from a risk management perspective. These include:

- What are the risk areas?
- What should the modification strategy be?
- How should the modification programme be designed?
  (1) Structure
  (2) Process
  (3) Outcome
  (4) Timescales
  (5) Resource utilisation.
- How will the Pathways project link into other trust/organisation/unit initiatives?
- Does the project definition report and project plan identify and analyse the risks for this project?
- How can the risks be avoided and contingency plans allowed for?

The risk modification cycle

The risk modification cycle (Fig. 13.3) is similar to the audit cycle and needs to cater for the needs of all staff providing care, the patients and their relatives and their ongoing support. The multi-disciplinary team can begin to apply risk management to their own health care setting, and achieve risk modification using this path as follows:

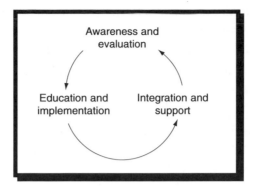

Fig. 13.3   The risk modification cycle.

(1) Awareness and evaluation

An in-depth assessment of the organisation's services and practices, and the costs relating to each, can begin to provide data on which potential risk areas can be identified. Included in this identification process are both the clinical and non-clinical components of the organisation that contribute to the overall episode of care. Awareness is the first phase of risk modification.

(2) Education and implementation

Development of processes and interventions that begin to change the undesirable practices of systems identified, is the second phase of risk modification. This combines specific structural and procedural changes to be implemented, with an educational process for all involved.

(3) Integration and support

Once changes and interventions are decided upon, a system for monitoring their integration into the organisation is needed to determine if the change has actually reduced or modified the identified risk. The data collection, analysis, measurement, monitoring and re-evaluation is the third part of risk modification.

A proactive risk modification process enables managers and the multi-disciplinary team to control effectively the safety, activity, cost and quality of health care service delivery. This can be linked into the Pathways of Care system, ensuring that changes in practices and hands-on care to patients are consistent, and variations reduced, thereby promoting appropriateness, effectiveness and efficiency.

The proactive risk modification process can be enhanced by carefully examining the different components of project management and the different steps of implementation and ongoing support, once the project moves to being accepted as part of everyday routine practice.

Risk identification

Producing a checklist to identify all areas of actual or potential risk can be most useful in the first step of the risk management process. The checklist questions below are aimed at helping the reader think about the Pathway project system, to identify potential risk areas.

The project environment

Project integration

- Is there a clear trust/organisational mission statement and objectives to which the project contributes?
- Is there consistency between the trust/organisation's existing strategic plans and the Pathway project?
- Will the Pathway project be integrated with other change management initiatives being introduced at the same time?
- Have the various initiatives been prioritised in recognition that the trust can only achieve change on a phased basis?

Trust/organisation cultural and management environment

- Will the existing culture and climate of opinion hinder the move to multi-disciplinary integration?
- Are working relationships between clinical staff and managers within the trust/organisation under strain?
- Are there sufficient clinical staff and managers with vision and motivation to lead their colleagues into successful multi-disciplinary integration and the formulation of Pathways of Care?
- Are all staff receptive to improving the quality of care delivery through analysis of variances, peer review and clinical audit?
- Is the trust/organisation's management style and the steering group's commitment suitable for the many demands of the Pathway project?

Project scope and a business case

- Has the Pathway project been fully endorsed and approved by the trust/organisation, board and the steering group?

- Is the size of this project significantly bigger than others the trust/organisation has tackled in the recent past?

Objectives and scope

- Are there clear project goals and objectives against which the Pathway project's success can be measured?
- Are there multi-disciplinary members involved to whom the scope of the Pathway project is unclear or confusing?

Benefits

- Have the benefits and success criteria been thought through and agreed?
- Is it clear what new care delivery methods, peer review and quality measures will be in place when the project has finished?
- Are there benefits and quality standards which can be measured?
- Is there a clearly defined mechanism to ensure that expected benefits are delivered?
- Does the project plan demonstrate how products will be delivered and the activities necessary to ensure they are delivered on time and to required quality standards?

Project planning

Method and approach

- Has a considered decision been taken about the use of a structured project management methodology or approach?
- Has the scope of the Pathway project been structured into the ward-level teams' activities?
- Are there identified objectives, deliverables and tasks for each Pathway diagnosis being considered?
- Have the Pathway steering group milestones been identified within the overall Pathway project?
- Is the trust/organisation sure about who is responsible for each deliverable?
- Are the roles and responsibilities for all the key stakeholders clearly identified?

Estimating and detailed planning

- Is there a clear Pathway project plan?

- Do detailed and complete stages of Pathway plans exist showing the sequence of the stages, their duration, multi-disciplinary team involvement and costs of each Pathway?
- Have detailed estimates been made of the quantity of work by all team members and the resource implications?
- Are estimates proving to be inaccurate as the project progresses?
- Is planning a continuous activity and are all the project plans up to date?
- Is feedback on progress against the plan easy to obtain?
- Are short-term targets set to maintain impetus?
- Is the timetable realistic and are deadlines achievable?

Project management structure

Project direction

- Is there a clearly identified project sponsor?
- Is the project sponsor fully supportive of and leading the project?
- Has the trust/organisation Pathway steering group been set up with clear terms of reference?
- Is the Pathway steering group useful in driving and guiding the project?

Project management

- Is there a project co-ordinator with the right level of skill and experience to manage effectively?
- Does the project co-ordinator have sufficient authority to manage all aspects of the project?
- Does the project co-ordinator have enough time dedicated to the project to manage it successfully?

Project execution

- Is there a Pathway steering group and ward-level teams with clearly defined roles and responsibilities?
- Is there a suitable appointed care manager for each Pathway, who is responsible for all the activities, variance collection and monitoring on a daily basis?
- Are multi-disciplinary team members with the necessary skills and experience committed to the project?
- Are all the necessary resources available to support the Pathway project to meet agreed timescales throughout the pilot period and during ongoing implementation?

- Will the data and information being collected be suitable for an option appraisal and determining the roll-out or cessation of the project?

Project control

- Is it clear where the Pathway project stands at any given time?
- Is there an effective way of getting decisions taken?
- Are there adequate progress monitoring and feedback mechanisms to keep the relevant people informed and to allow early correction of problems?

Change management

- Do formal procedures exist to handle project issues and problems?
- If so, are they effective?
- Do change control procedures exist which manage changes to the scope of the project?
- If so, are they effective?

Quality management

- Are there quality objectives or standards for the things the Pathway project is to produce?
- Are there appropriate quality assurance procedures to review the quality of all the Pathway project products?
- Are quality checkpoints and reviews built into the project plan?

Acceptance within the trust/organisation

- Is the Pathway project clearly understood and endorsed by clinical staff and managers?
- Do the relevant managers know and agree the timescales by which they will start to obtain benefit from the Pathway project?
- Are some staff reluctant to undertake the changes necessary for successful implementation?
- Do staff appreciate the extent and necessity for education and training?

Next steps

Once the checklist is complete, the level of concern is rated as causing 'more concern' or 'less concern', then ranked in order of the probability of the risk occurring, and the amount of damage each would cause to the Pathway project if it occurred. The actions which will either eliminate the risk or reduce its impact are then agreed.

By using this process, you will have taken positive action for risk management. The next components of risk management should then be applied:

(1)   Risk analysis
(2)   Risk avoidance
(3)   Contingency planning.

Risk analysis

Having identified the possible risks, assess the probability of each risk occurring and estimate the impact. If nothing were done to counteract this risk, what impact would it have on the Pathway project?

This provides a clear focus of the risks and enables the steering group to concentrate on preventive action and contingency planning.

Risk avoidance

Develop risk reduction and prevention plans and build these into the Pathway project plan, asking the following questions:

- What action can be taken now to prevent this risk from happening?
- What action can be taken now to reduce the impact of this risk should it occur?
- Is the expense and time element of the preventive action preferable to the risk impact?

Action should be expressed in terms of time and cost. For example, extra education and training required costing £Z per head, for a team of 20 personnel, would entail a total cost of $20 \times £Z$.

Contingency planning

Where the risk could have severe consequences it is necessary to prepare contingency plans. Ask the question, 'If the risk does occur, what action would put the Pathway project back on track?'. While not preventing all the negative impact of the risk, a realistic contingency plan will enable the Pathway project to get back on track with minimum disruption to the overall plan. In order to maximise the chances of a contingency plan succeeding the following actions must be taken:

- If additional resources are required to implement the plans, arrangements should be made for them to be available at short notice

- Members of the Pathway steering group and ward-level teams must understand the plan and their role in it
- If the feasibility of the contingency plan is in any doubt it must, if possible, be tested

Risk identification and management should continue throughout the Pathway project for enhanced success.

Conclusion

To continuously improve the clinical process quality, reduce risk and appropriately control costs it is essential to eliminate inappropriate variation and document continuous improvement. Improving communication and documentation are fundamental to implementing a risk management system. This is exactly what Pathways of Care are all about and their usage is increasing both nationally and internationally. Health care research both in the UK (Ovretveit 1992) and USA (Berwick 1989) has demonstrated that it is process not people that make a system breakdown. Pathways are an excellent way of improving the integrated care process, facilitating system improvements which are key to increased quality and productivity, and the reduction of risk and unit costs. Effective co-ordination and management of the implementation of Pathways to a health care organisation is crucial to the overall success of moving from a pilot project to everyday practice. The most successful Pathway implementation sites are those with a dedicated Pathway co-ordinator who can provide direction, support and overall strategy to the use of Pathways.

From a risk management perspective Pathways are an effective risk management tool which can form the key direction of an overall risk organisational system, improving clinical practice and outcomes, and decreasing hospital liability. The main triad of a clinical risk modification programme in any health care system is guidelines, education and data. Pathways of Care encompass and continually use all three. Pathways provide a framework giving greater quality assurance in a timely way, with uniform quality, multi-disciplinary standards, and focus on continually learning from and improving upon the care delivery process.

References

Berwick, D. (1989) Continuous quality improvements in healthcare. *Journal of Nursing Quality Assurance*, August.
Deming, W.E. (1982) Quality, productivity and competitive position. MIT Centre for Advanced Engineering Study, Cambridge, Mass.

DoH (1993) *Improving Clinical Effectiveness*. EL(93)115. HMSO, London.

Ovretveit, J. (1992) *Quality Health Services*. Organisational and Social Studies, Brunel Institute, London.

Swage, T. & Wilson, J.H. (1995) Multidisciplinary pathways of care series: the purchaser's perspective. *Health Care Risk report*, October.

Thomson, R., Lavender, M. & Madhok, R. (1995) How to ensure guidelines are effective. *British Medical Journal*, 311, 22nd July.

Wilson, J.H. (1992) *An Introduction to Multidisciplinary Pathways of Care*, December. Report from Northern Regional Health Authority.

Information in this chapter appears in

Wilson, J. (ed.) (1996) *Integrated Care Management: The Path to Success?* Butterworth-Heinemann, Oxford.

Chapter 14

Pathways as a Basis for Evidence-based Contracting

Jenny Thornton

Introduction

In 1989/90 a government white paper heralded some fundamental changes to the way in which health care provision in Britain was organised. The 'purchaser provider split' separated the role of service provider from that of purchasers of services for defined populations. Managed units were invited to apply for trust status which offered service providers the opportunity to manage their own resources and gave them a certain amount of freedom and flexibility with regard to capital developments and marketing within the NHS framework.

Services are now purchased on behalf of a defined population by a wide range of purchasers. These include health agencies and general practitioner fund holders (GPFHs) who have been granted legislative authority to commission the purchasing of specified services under the NHS and Community Care Act 1990.

This act introduced an 'internal market' within the NHS that took effect in April 1991. It required purchasers of health care to negotiate contracts with providers, to meet the needs of the local resident population. Over the past few years this has promoted fierce competition between providers within the NHS.

Until recently the majority of purchasers have tended to purchase health care by means of a 'block contract': an agreed sum of money is given to a provider in return for a specified level of activity such as 'cases taken off the waiting list' or 'number of attendances'. This type of contract provides the purchaser with little or no information regarding the case-mix of clients, i.e. the type and severity of presentation of cases, or of the complexity of assessment and treatment required to meet the identified need.

Purchasers, especially GPFHs holding smaller budgets with less flexibility, feel that complex services such as departments of child and adolescent psychiatry are 'expensive'. Both the health agencies and GPFHs are unhappy with the limited information provided by block contracts and are steadily moving towards pricing structures which more accurately reflect the complexity of treatments offered in particular cases, with contracts such as 'cost and volume' and 'cost per case'. These types of contract help them retain flexibility to move funds quickly between providers, allowing both patient choice and value for money. However, from the provider's point of view, this generates a risk for trusts striving to secure their annual income from the variety of purchasers.

GPFHs within the NHS are gaining increasing purchasing power due to the development of the GPFH scheme. Their ability to contract outside their local area if acceptable information and pricing structures are not forthcoming locally is motivating providers to drive the process of costed care packages to support an evidence-based contracting process.

All purchasers are increasingly scrutinising their contracts in terms of what they get for their money. They are demanding that the contracts be broken down to allow money to follow the client. The price of contracts for care must therefore accurately reflect the complexity of intervention for a particular client. At present, pricing structures within NHS trusts are often based on inadequate information. As trusts are required to secure more and more of their contracted income on a 'cost per case' basis, they are running a significant financial risk of not recovering the income they require.

Purchasers continually strive to commission high quality healthcare within the limited resources available. It is essential that they have a good knowledge of the needs of their population to enable them to develop long term purchasing strategies. It is equally important that they are given comprehensive information regarding the components of service provision and anticipated outcomes of treatment by service providers, to support these purchasing strategies and ensure both value for money and clinical effectiveness.

Traditionally it has been difficult to identify and quantify the outcomes of many healthcare interventions due to the unpredictability of treatments, the diversity of individual client needs and the lack of research and evaluation studies available. This lack of information is a handicap for providers attempting to justify the relatively high prices of more complex service provision and is one of the strongest arguments for the investment by providers in the costed care package methodology for supporting evidence-based contracting.

This chapter sets out one method of introducing evidence-based contracts using Pathways of Care to support the process.

The costed care package philsophy

When seeking to develop an evidence-based contract framework, it is important that the objectives for its introduction be clearly agreed with

clinicians, managers, purchasers and providers. Full involvement of all
these parties is necessary to map out the information flows required to
establish the care packages.

Objectives may include the provision of management information to
support contract monitoring by the purchasers related to activity and cost,
the development of a method for analysing the financial effects of potential
changes in activity and case-mix, and the evaluation of the costs of operating
different care packages. In addition, clinicians may wish to include objectives relating to the setting and monitoring of standards related to the best
clinical practice for an average client, within a defined client group.

To enable these objectives to be achieved, historical data is required
regarding case-mix, types and complexities of treatments offered and
activity levels within previous block contracts.

Providers need to identify exactly what services they aim to provide, how
they will be provided and to agree expected outcomes. This process will
give a focused approach to care and will help with the planning of a long
term strategic direction for the provider.

The costed care package framework has two aspects. The first relates to
the information and structure of the care package, and the second to the
costing.

The development of care packages

'Care package' is the term used to describe the combination of interventions
that a client receives as part of their care.

Although individual care packages are tailored to meet the needs of
particular clients, it is helpful to define clients into 'target groups' in order
to agree protocols or guidelines for care packages which ensure best clinical
practice. In order to develop these packages it is necessary to undertake a
number of tasks (Fig. 14.1). Some of the terminology will not be familiar to
the reader as it has been developed to support the care package process. Full
explanations of each term follow, together with a detailed description of
each task.

Analysis of activity for a service

The first step in developing care packages for a particular service is to
identify the target group(s) to which the care packages will relate. It is
therefore necessary to make an analysis of the patterns of referral to the
service over recent years in order to identify the type, number and
percentage of referrals. Forecasts of likely future activity are then made,
upon which to base future costings.

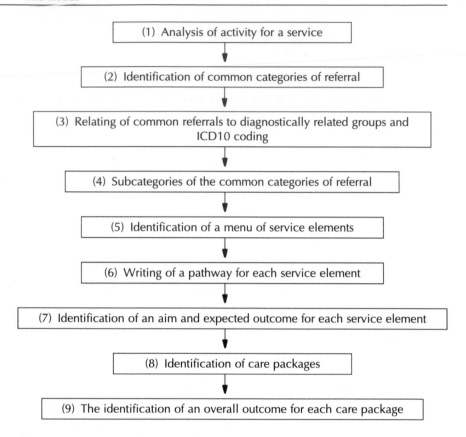

Fig. 14.1 The process for developing care packages in child and adolescent psychiatry.

Identification of common categories of referral

From the analysis of referrals made to the service, it is possible to establish a set of common categories of referral: a list of common conditions for which clients are referred to that service. Referrers should be able to recognise these categories as those for which they would refer clients to that service, as it is these categories which will relate to the menu of care packages (Fig. 14.2).

Relating of common referrals to diagnostically related groups and ICD10 coding

Having identified the common categories of referral to the service, it is then possible to relate these categories to diagnostically related groups (DRGs)

- Behavioural problems
- Emotional problems
- Overdose/self harm
- Eating disorders

Fig. 14.2   Examples of common categories of referral.

and, in the department of child and adolescent psychiatry, to the associated discharge (ICD10) codes (Table 14.1). This breakdown will support research, particularly in relation to the evaluation of outcomes.

Subcategories of the common categories of referral

For the purpose of tailoring care packages to meet the wide range of clients' needs, it is necessary to subcategorise each common category of referral. In the example of the department of child and adolescent psychiatry, each common category of referral is banded by age group and severity (Table 14.2).

Identification of a menu of service elements

The term 'service element' refers to an individual component of service provision which can be offered as part of a comprehensive care package. For ease of use it is helpful to list the various service elements under sub-headings.

In the department of child and adolescent psychiatry, the service elements are identified and categorised under the following headings:

Table 14.1   Example of a diagnostically related group (DRG) with ICD10 coding.

ICD10 code	Diagnostically related group	ICD10 subcode	Diagnostically related group description
F91	Conduct disorders	F91.0	Conduct disorder confined to the family context
		F91.1	Unsocialised conduct disorder
		F91.2	Socialised conduct disorder
		F91.3	Oppositional defiant disorder
		F91.8	Other conduct disorders
		F91.9	Conduct disorder, unspecified

Table 14.2 Example of the sub-categorisation of a common category of referral.

Common category of referral	Age band	Severity
Behavioural problems	Preschool	Mild Moderate Severe
	School age	Mild Moderate Severe
	Adolescent	Mild Moderate Severe

(1)   Pre-assessment (from the referral of a case to the allocation of that case to a clinician)
(2)   Assessment
(3)   Out-patient treatment
(4)   Day unit treatment
(5)   Consultation, liaison, advice and training
(6)   Medication and supervision of medication
(7)   Discharge

Examples of service elements listed under out-patient treatments include:

• Behaviour family treatment (incorporating parent management training and/or behaviour modification and/or parent child game) – part I, brief
• Behaviour family treatment (incorporating parent management training and/or behaviour modification and/or parent child game) – part II, routine
• Behaviour family treatment (incorporating parent management training and/or behaviour modification and/or parent child game) – part III, complex
• Brief intervention service
• Attention training for attention deficit hyperactivity disorder

Writing of a Pathway for each service element

Once all the service elements for a particular service have been identified, Pathways are written for each one. Each Pathway describes the best agreed clinical practice for that component of service. It includes measurable standards in both the administrative and clinical areas and, where appropriate, measures of clinical effectiveness such as developmental inventories, behaviour checklists and problem rating scales. Satisfaction questionnaires for the client, staff and referrer can also be built into the Pathways.

Identification of an aim and expected outcome for each service element

An aim and expected outcome are identified for each service element. The recording of these for each Pathway serves a number of purposes. Clear aims focus the attention of the clinician on the specific use of an intervention and help to clarify outcome expectations with the client and the referrer. In addition, the collation of the information over time will aid the development and use of interventions which demonstrate good outcomes.

Identification of care packages

With the menu of service elements and the common categories of referral agreed for the service, the next task is to decide which service elements should form the basic care package for each subcategory of the common categories of referral. Likely additional service elements are listed separately and relate to components of service provision which are only sometimes offered for clients within that category of referral, according to individual need.

Mapping out all the conditions likely to be referred to a service and the likely response in terms of service delivery to each of these target groups, offers the provider a powerful information tool for marketing, supervision, teaching and induction. It also provides the information required to cost the various service components and to monitor contracts.

The identification of an overall outcome for each care package

This stage of the care package process is probably the most ambitious and is currently the subject of a great deal of research and discussion, particularly in relation to the more complex cases seen. For example, in the field of community mental health, the identification of anticipated outcomes for defined target groups following an agreed care package is very difficult. However, by attempting to agree outcomes under the headings of 'client-related', 'clinician-related' and 'referrer-related', we have found it possible to monitor them over time, gaining experience which will help refine the future prediction of outcomes. It will take many years before a service has sufficient data upon which to base realistic and acceptable outcome predictions.

The costing of care packages

The second aspect of the care package framework relates to costing of the care packages. Pathways are built into the contracting process and a price established for each category of referral through the costing of each Pathway. As with the development of the care packages themselves, it is necessary to undertake a series of tasks (Fig. 14.3).

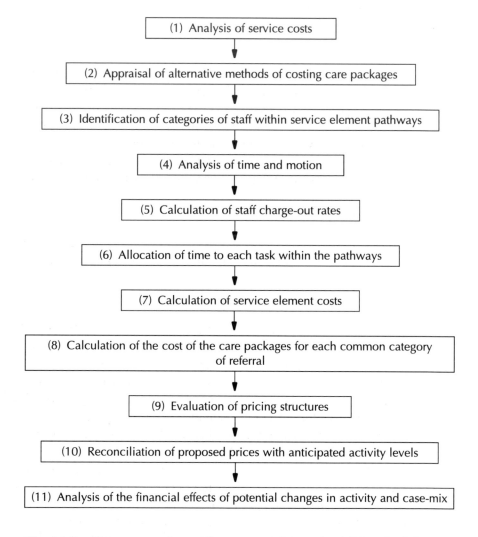

Fig. 14.3   The process for costing care packages in child and adolescent psychiatry.

Analysis of service costs

Before appraising appropriate methods of costing care packages, it is necessary to establish a full, accurate and current cost of the service.

Direct costs

The direct costs of a service are obtained from the service budgets, categorised into pay and non-pay expenditure. Pending pay awards are also taken into account.

Indirect costs

Indirect costs relating to a service are calculated to include the gross salaries (including all 'on-costs' e.g. employer's National Insurance) of the appropriate managers. These costs are allocated to the various parts of the service on the basis of whole time equivalents (w.t.e.s) as this is likely to be the determining factor in the allocation of their workload.

Other indirect costs such as domestic services, estate and telephone expenditure are allocated on the basis of the floor area used by the service.

Overhead costs

Overhead expenditure such as finance and human resource department costs are apportioned on the basis of direct plus indirect expenditure.

Appraisal of alternative methods of costing care packages

NHS Management Executive (NHSME) guidance FDL(93)59, *Costing for Contracting – The 1994/5 Contracting Round*, states that prices should be set at full cost with no planned cross-subsidisation between services. Therefore, income received by the provider's services should match the full cost of these services. There are numerous accounting techniques which can be used to achieve this goal. The method described is a 'top down/bottom up' costing process and is given to illustrate the philosophy rather than as a strict template for others to follow.

Whatever the costing methodology used, in order to attribute a price to each common category of referral, it is necessary to calculate the cost of each service element and then collate these costs into the various care packages. Indirect and overhead costs are apportioned to each of the service elements and then allocated to the target groups. The bottom-up technique incorporates 'activity-based costing' whereby staff costs represent a cost pool, and staff input into each service element pathway represents the 'cost driver'.

Identification of categories of staff within service element pathways

The Pathways written for each service element are used as a basis for costing by detailing the grade of staff and the time taken for each activity set out in the Pathway. The main cost driver in each Pathway is staff time. To ease the costings, staff grades are collated into categories (Table 14.3).

Table 14.3   Categories of staff within service element Pathways.

Category of staff	Grade of staff
Consultant	Consultant
Higher clinical	Principal clinical psychologist Behavioural nurse specialist Senior I therapists
Lower clinical	Lower grade clinical staff
Administration	Secretarial staff of all grades

Analysis of time and motion

A 'charge-out' rate is required for each category of staff to apply to the timed tasks set out in the Pathways. The calculation of a charge-out rate gives a 'cost per Pathway minute' for each category of staff and takes account of time spent on indirect patient-related and non patient-related activity, such as training and meetings which are not recorded on the Pathways.

In order to calculate this charge-out rate, all clinical and administration staff are required to undertake a time and motion study over a four week period. The format of this study is designed separately for clinical and administrative staff, to reflect their different roles and tasks.

In the particular time and motion study designed by the Hounslow and Spelthorne department of child and adolescent psychiatry, time was broken down so that one unit represented six minutes, which allowed easy calculations to be made based on ten units per hour. It was also designed in a way which enabled staff to record interruptions alongside ongoing tasks. This made the task of recording activities against time more straightforward for staff, whilst allowing accurate times for each activity to be calculated during the final stages of analysis.

The results of the time and motion study are then used to calculate a 'percentage time per staff' category spent on 'direct Pathway-related activities' which can be related to the tasks contained within the Pathways (Table 14.4).

Table 14.4   Examples of direct Pathway related activities that can be related to the tasks contained in a Pathway.

Staff group	Direct pathway-related activities
Clinical staff	Face to face client contacts Telephone discussions with clients Dictation, report writing and reading client notes Liaison meetings and case conferences
Administrative staff	Typing of client reports Typing of letters and sending of appointments

Calculation of staff charge-out rates

The charge-out rate per minute is calculated for each member of staff as shown in Table 14.5, and then averaged into each of the various staff categories.

Allocation of time to each task within the Pathways

In order to attribute a cost to each Pathway, it is necessary to analyse each Pathway in terms of the category of staff undertaking each task set out in the Pathway and the expected time it would take to complete each task. This needs to be agreed for each Pathway by the clinical and administrative staff who routinely complete the tasks.

Table 14.5   Fictitious example of the calculation of a 'charge-out rate' for a member of staff.

Name	w.t.e	Hours worked per week	% Week spent on 'direct activities'	Weeks worked per annum	Hours worked on 'direct activities' per annum	Gross salary per annum [£]	Average cost per hour [£]	Charge-out rate per minute [£]
xxx	1.00	36	64%	43.2	995.3	15 648	15.27	0.25

Calculation of service element costs

From the analysis of staff time within each Pathway, it is then possible to calculate the cost of each service element by multiplying the total number of minutes for each of the categories of staff by their individual charge-out rates. Once the service element costs are reconciled to the service budget, a percentage is applied to these direct costs to enable indirect and overhead costs to be recovered.

Calculation of the cost of the care packages for each common category of referral

In order to calculate the cost of each common category of referral, it is necessary to add together the costs of the individual service elements which together form the basic care package for each of the categories. The likely additional service elements for each of the common categories of referral are priced separately in line with the care package philosophy discussed earlier in the chapter (Fig. 14.4).

Evaluation of pricing structures

Various accounting techniques can be used to determine pricing structures. Three obvious frameworks include:

(1) A detailed price list for each subcategory of the common categories of referral by basic care package and likely additional service elements
(2) A detailed price list for each subcategory of the common categories of referral, which takes into account the average combination of basic care package and likely additional service elements in each case
(3) A list of prices collated into several 'bands'

The first option poses the highest risk to the provider in terms of the necessary reconciliation of income back to the service. However, it is likely to be the most popular pricing framework from the point of view of a purchaser as they will only be required to pay for the care actually provided to the individual client(s).

The second option is also likely to be acceptable to purchasers who will be able to plan their annual expenditure based on any information they may have available about their expected type and number of referrals over a one year period. Regular evaluation and feedback, both within providers and to purchasers and referrers relating to the accuracy of these assumptions about the likely average combination of service elements making up each care

**Example of a costed care package
for one category of referral**

Element of care package	Example	
Common referral	Autism	
ICD10 Code	F84	
Age group	Pre-school	
Severity/complexity	Severe	
Basic care package	HA9:	Autistic disorder pre-assessment
	HB11:	Autistic/asperger syndrome complex assessment
	HC22:	Social development team treatment Programme for children with autism or autistic-like syndromes
	HE1:	Consultation with other professionals/ agencies – by telephone
	HE4:	Network and review meeting – convened by the department of child and adolescent psychiatry – by telephone
	HF2:	Medication and supervision of medication
	HG1:	General discharge package
Cost of basic care package	£1000	
Likely additional service elements	HE5:	Network and review meeting – convened by another agency – at another base
	HB14:	Medical examination
Costs of each additional service element	HE5:	£100
	HB14:	£120

Fig. 14.4 A costed care package for autism from Hounslow and Spelthorne Community and Mental Health NHS Trust.

package, will enable the ongoing refinement of more accurate care profiles and will further inform the contracting process.

The third of the three pricing structures simplifies invoicing but loses some of the accuracy of the costings.

Particularly in the early stages of introducing evidence-based contracting based on costed care packages, providers will probably lack detailed, accurate information about historical referral and service patterns. They will probably therefore wish to minimise the risk related to the securing of their annual income, and to launch the new model using the third, banded pricing structure. This is also a sensible choice if the price differences between the various common categories of referral are not too great.

Another issue which must be considered when developing a pricing structure for the evidence-based contracting framework is the resource implications in terms of the staff time and information technology systems required to support the collection, collation and invoicing of these complex pricing structures. The need for a computerised database to support the process is further discussed later in the chapter.

Reconciliation of proposed prices with anticipated activity levels

When considering the risk to a provider of launching a new pricing framework, it is imperative that the care package prices are set at a level that will recover the full costs of the services, whilst not over-pricing them. To undertake this reconciliation it is necessary to establish the expected activity levels for each common category of referral per annum.

As described earlier in the chapter, a detailed analysis of activity is necessary to establish the numbers and patterns of referrals to the service. These referrals are then broken down into the common categories of referral identified as part of the Pathway process, and a weighted average percentage of each category is calculated. This percentage is then applied to the overall target activity figures for the service. By multiplying the individual prices for each of the common categories of referral by the activity levels described above, the predicted income recovery can be compared to the full cost of providing the service, to ensure that the costs are recovered.

Providers may also be interested in calculating whether this level of care package is achievable within current staffing resources. This is done by multiplying the hours for each category of staff in each care package by the overall target activity profile for that service. Most providers will find that this raises interesting questions relating to their contracted activity levels. It is recognised that current activity levels in many areas of the NHS rely heavily upon staff working additional hours of unpaid over-time and on short-cuts to planned delivery of care or recording of information.

Analysis of the financial effects of potential changes in activity and case-mix

Once the spreadsheet necessary for the calculations described above has been set up, it is possible to undertake a number of other calculations and analyses to support a flexible evidence-based contracting process and to facilitate the planning of services for the future.

The total costs of a service are comprised of direct, indirect and overhead expenditure. These costs can be further categorised into variable, semi-fixed and fixed elements. Variable costs can be defined as costs which increase in response to an increase in activity. Semi-fixed costs remain fixed over a range of activity, but increase when particular volumes of activity are reached. Fixed costs are independent of activity and so remain constant. For example, clinical and administrative staff costs can be defined as semi-fixed costs as additional staff are usually only required for a major change in activity. Consultants, however, are defined as fixed costs as services rarely require additional consultants as activity increases. Taking these definitions into account, calculations can be made to determine the effect on prices of any potential changes in activity and case-mix.

Need for a client-centred, computerised information system to support the evidence-based contracting process

In order for costed care packages to drive the evidence based contracting process, it is essential that the information collected around client-related activity is recorded onto a system which can not only store it, but also manipulate the information to produce useful reports. This is particularly important when considering the time taken by clinicians to record all the information necessary to support the care package process. Clinicians are required to record the following:

(1) The categorisation of each client in relation to a common category of referral
(2) The selected combination of service elements for each individual client
(3) The completion of Pathways for each service element undertaken, including the full and accurate recording of variances
(4) The focused approach to patient care and service delivery required by the use of the 'problem, goal, plan and notes' recording system
(5) Various outcomes for each service element undertaken and for each common category of referral.

It is essential that clinicians are given adequate training and support, both in the use of Pathways and the recording of service element activity, in order to ensure a uniform approach to classification and recording.

The entering of selected information onto a client-centered database will:

(1) Enable comparison between 'actual' and 'expected' care package delivery for each common category of referral
(2) Enable the long term evaluation and refining of service delivery
(3) Build up an information database related to all aspects of client care to support clinical research and benchmarking
(4) Facilitate the sharing of information and the co-ordination of care across the multi-disciplinary teams
(5) Enable the generation of the minimum data set and information needed for the raising of invoices

Variances recorded in Pathways are still manually collected and collated to enable the following:

(1) Comparison between 'agreed best practice' and 'actual practice'
(2) Monitoring of standards
(3) Scrutinisation of deviations from expected care both for each individual client and for each common category of referral, to identify trends and patterns of service delivery

Conclusion

Wherever costed care packages are introduced it will be important to evaluate whether the care package prices are sustainable in the marketplace. GPFHs are particularly influenced by price comparisons as their purchasing is increasingly undertaken on a cost per case basis.

Demand for costed care packages will also be affected by the long term purchasing strategies of individual purchasers and of the NHS as a whole. The development of competition within the NHS and the need to meet the information requirements of the various purchasers will also encourage the development of costed care packages.

Information regarding the cost of services ensures value for money and allows the re-evaluation of expensive areas of service provision. Knowledge about the behaviour of these costs is essential for the planning of service developments and for assessing the impact on services of resource cuts. This identification and describing of the services offered increases the information available to providers for the education and marketing of services to purchasers.

The development and costing of care packages places services in a stronger position to face the increased competition offered by the new internal market and the expansion of the GPFH scheme. Whilst care packages do not offer treatments at a lower price, the prices do reflect the complexity of treatments involved and state an expected treatment outcome. This body of information can then be used to underpin the contracting process and to enable purchasers and providers to make informed decisions with regard to planning their future strategies.

Chapter 15

Automation of Pathways

Garry Favor and Rebecca Ricks

Introduction

Although the practice of case management, using manual Pathways of Care, critical paths, or Care Maps®, has made major contributions in improving patient care and lowering cost, its benefits will remain limited without automation. The benefits to be obtained through automation depend on a health care organisation's status in the development of their case management programme. Automation can involve several levels from simply building and printing Pathways, to collecting and entering variances into a computerised database for trending and analysis, to full automation of Pathways with integrated documentation by all care providers. In order to install a fully integrated Pathway documentation system, an organisation must have a major commitment to the process and must have made significant progress in implementing a manual programme. A process cannot be automated if it is not understood.

This chapter will provide information on four levels of automation for case management, and will review what can be provided at each level. This will include expected benefits, automation requirements and limitations. The ultimate goal of Pathway automation is a fully integrated documentation system in which variances are collected automatically as clinicians chart their care. The data is coded as it is entered, making rules-based decision support as well as trending and analysis reporting possible. What is involved in developing and implementing such a system will be reviewed, as well as progress to date on achieving this level of automation. Finally, there will be a look at the future of automation with the possibility of real time decision alerts concerning possible variances, and automated case management workstations with on-line data reporting and graphing of current and past patient populations.

Limitations of a manual process

The primary limitation to a manual process is the large amount of data collected which needs to be analysed and evaluated daily for individual patient care, as well as combining the outcomes of multiple patients to determine possible system process improvements. Clinicians of all disciplines are overloaded with data in today's partially automated environment. Laboratory results, procedure results and clinical observations are flooding care givers moment by moment. What are the critical pieces? How do clinicians put information together, such as a laboratory test result, a clinical observation, and a drug dose as they sort through reams of clinical documentation recorded in multiple areas of the patient record? It is no wonder, despite all efforts to improve processes, define care requirements and streamline report mechanisms, that catastrophic mistakes continue to be made in patient care, and what might appear as obvious solutions under other circumstances, are never identified and implemented.

With the obvious need for automation, why does health care continue to lag behind other businesses in achieving automated solutions? A recent survey of chief information officers in the USA found that health care organisations were investing record amounts of their capital dollars and increasing the operating budgets of their information systems (IS) departments to achieve integrated health systems (HIMSS/HP Survey 1995). If improvements in current documentation processes are not also provided, patient care will benefit from this effort to only a limited degree. Health care organisations need to identify and incorporate solutions that improve their current care processes, not just their information network. It is not enough to automate today's manual patient care system. The goal must be to push beyond where we are today to tomorrow's information solutions.

Health care organisations are having to spend increasing amounts of their clinicians' time trying to collect patient data and organise it into some kind of meaningful presentation. This task continues to absorb more and more of the patient care provider's time, yet it does not meaningfully contribute to improved patient care; rather it takes the clinician away from the patient. Physicians are becoming increasingly frustrated with today's manual and automated documentation efforts and with little wonder. Ancillary laboratory, radiology, therapy, pharmacy, and nursing information systems provide a wealth of data, none of which is truly integrated or presented to the doctor in such a way that sense can easily be made of it. But if data is recorded somewhere in the chart and the physician fails to put it together with other relevant data, no matter how daunting the task, he/she is then potentially at fault if a poor patient outcome results.

This then is the task to which case management automation efforts are directed. Manual Pathways of Care help direct the clinician's efforts in providing patient care and evaluating the results against the expected outcomes. This has helped to improve the chaos of tracking a patient's care in today's health care system, but automation is critical to managing the volumes of data which need to be tracked in order to improve and document patient outcomes.

Four levels of automation

Automation can provide assistance in the case management process at four levels (Fig. 15.1). The highest level is where the greatest benefit to clinicians and patients can be achieved.

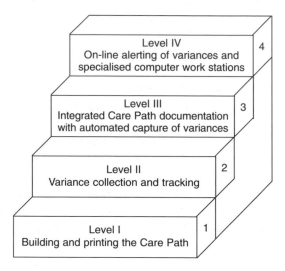

Fig. 15.1   The steps towards achieving the automated care path documentation system.

The lowest level with the least benefits is automating the ability to build Pathways and print them for manual documentation. The second level is the ability to enter variances retrospectively into a database for all patients on predefined Pathways and then providing reports for trending and analysis to make Pathway improvements. The third level is complete automation of Pathways with integrated documentation, in which variances are captured automatically as charting takes place. Clinicians of all disciplines will benefit from this effort by having immediate access to this information. The documentation should be collected in such a manner that it is automatically coded so that trending and analysis reporting for groups of patients can be performed months and years later. The potential benefits from such a system will revolutionise patient care.

The fourth level is where the real benefits of automation can result. It is the ability to provide on-line decision support for potential variances, and on-line reporting and graphing of individual and multiple patient outcomes concurrently rather than retrospectively.

Level 1 – building and printing Pathways of Care

The first requirement by nearly all organisations when starting their Pathway programme is a quick, user friendly method to simply build and print Pathways for manual documentation. These manual Pathways of Care can be presented to a multi-disciplinary team for review and approval. They can also be used by multiple clinicians, including physicians, to document what actually transpired in the patient's care and where variances occurred. Because there is usually only one copy of the manual Pathway for a patient, there are sometimes practical problems with many disciplines using it to record care at the same time. These practical considerations involve the location of the Pathway and the need to keep it streamlined for easy review.

Of particular interest to new Pathway programmes is the ability to build their manual Pathways cheaply and to modify them easily. As manual Pathways are initially developed and put into use, there are many changes made to them on a frequent basis. Revising Pathways can be a tedious and time consuming process in a manual environment.

Most vendors of computer facilities are not investing in the development of software simply to build and print Pathways for manual documentation and review. This is probably due to several factors. One reason vendors may not be interested in this market is the failure to standardise the Pathway format across organisations. Any review of Pathways from different organisations will show wide variation in how they are laid out. This makes it difficult for vendors to develop software and graphical print-outs to suit such a wide ranging market. In addition, most organisations have adapted some other form of software to accomplish this task, albeit with less than completely satisfactory results.

Many Pathway users when asked, will admit to using some type of word processing or a spreadsheet application to build their Pathways. Other organisations use typesetting by a print shop to produce manual Pathways. Use of some form of software to build and print Pathways has the advantage of relatively fast turn around time for modifications (although they are not always easy to make) and less expense incurred when compared to print shops. Some organisations have adapted the document building software of their hospital information system to print the Pathways automatically. This usually involves so-called 'hard coding', meaning that the document must be completely rebuilt, usually by the IS department, every time a modification must be made to it. This too is an expensive and time consuming method of generating manual Pathways of Care.

Although paper-based Pathways do help an organisation guide the care for predefined case types, they have several limitations. One is that the variance data recorded must be manually collected from the forms and tabulated or entered into a computer data base for trending and analysis. Needless to say this is a time consuming process with less than accurate results. Another limitation sometimes encountered is fragmentation between the manual Pathway and other clinical documentation, which makes it difficult for a clinician to see the full picture and accurately identify all potential variances that are occurring.

Very often in current manual environments, there is also a great deal of redundant documentation. Clinicians may be documenting against a manual Pathway and also recording the same information on graphic forms, flow sheets, observation charts or in notes. A final limitation to paper Pathways is the inability to easily customise them to an individual patient. To modify the Pathway, clinicians must manually add to a map, complete a variance tracking form, or strike through inappropriate interventions or outcomes. The clinicians may even have to write out a new plan of care using a blank form for patients that fall off the Pathway or fail to progress as planned. Because of the limitations in the use of manual Pathways, as well as the variations in layout, it is not likely that vendors of computer equipment will develop software simply to build and print Pathways of Care.

Level 2 – variance collection and tracking

It is at the second level of automation – variance collection and tracking – that several vendors are entering the market. This software provides for data entry of variances that are collected in a manual environment. The variances are usually entered into a database by a data processing clerk, case manager, or automated image reader technology.

The benefits to such software include the ability to collect a variety of data for trending and analysis reporting. Depending on the software, the data elements collected can be very few or they can be extensive. The variety and depth of the trending and analysis reports provided depends on the software product. A product that allows for easy modification and building of reports (such as a menu selection of data elements), will certainly provide more benefit to a programme than software that has the capability for only a limited number of prebuilt reports. Such data collection systems must be easy to learn and easy to use for data entry and retrieval. These systems give clinicians a good start to collecting and analysing variance data for identifying problem areas and making improvements to Pathways and patient care.

The limitations of such software are readily apparent. They are 'stand alone' systems requiring a great deal of time to collect and enter the pertinent data. In some cases they may have data entry limitations, such as the failure to provide data fields for cost and risk factors. These limitations usually occur because clinicians helping to design such systems do not realise the need for these additional data elements. The systems are also limited in their reporting capability. There is usually good general report capability provided, but the ability to do complicated statistical analysis may not be available.

Also, the systems may not have the provision for truly focused reporting capability when possible trends are suspected. An example of this need for focused reporting might be that a case manager notices that the patients on a particular Pathway are not mobilising as expected following surgery. The case manager would probably want to create a special, focused report that listed all of the patients who failed to mobilise when expected, along with most common other variances that were occurring at the same time. This might reveal that the next most common variance being recorded is treatment for nausea and vomiting. This would help to identify that nausea was the most likely cause of the patients failing to mobilise as expected. With such information the case manager could review with the pharmacists, physicians and anaesthetists what changes should be made in the Pathway to achieve the desired outcome. Without the ability to create such focused reports these trends can be difficult to identify or confirm.

Level 3 – integrated Pathways of Care documentation systems

When automating Pathways of Care for clinical documentation, there are several considerations. Many organisations have made their manual Pathways part of their charting documentation system. This encourages greater usage by clinicians and ensures better tracking of variances. One of the problems with this is that it may add to the charting process for clinicians already overloaded by documentation requirements, if the Pathway does not replace current paperwork. In addition, most organisations usually have multiple speciality stand alone information systems for areas such as the intensive care unit, the accident and emergency department, and therapy care settings.

The data collected on these different systems does not flow together, and computer interfaces are not only expensive but the data is often mismatched. Many current hospital information systems are fragmented along the same lines as a manual chart. A clinician must follow one path for current orders, another for laboratory and radiology results, still another to see the care plan, and another to view progress notes. This kind of fragmentation not only increases the documentation load of clinicians but it also frustrates their attempts to bring the variety of clinical data together. Moving from computer screen to computer screen is even more tedious than going from page to page of a manual chart. Clinicians are demanding that their systems be integrated, that data collected be available wherever needed, and that the system should flow logically and with ease.

The development of such a system involves careful evaluation of the data collection process as well as a clear understanding of the expected benefits and problems that may be encountered. System requirements can then be determined. An organisation that installs a system such as this, which so drastically changes the current process, must also understand the commitment required to support the users after implementation in order to ensure long term success. The change process involved in replacing manual systems with such dramatic automation efforts cannot be underestimated and requires a shared vision and commitment at all levels of an organisation, from the executive to the physicians to middle management and the end users. It is at the critical point of installation and the first six to twelve months following implementation, that many such efforts will be undermined and fail, despite large investments of capital and resources for the planning, development, and installation of the product.

We now focus on several aspects of developing and implementing an integrated Pathway documentation system, starting with a discussion concerning the importance of data collection. We will then review limitations to current development efforts. The expected benefits from integrating Pathways of Care and clinical documentation will follow. System requirements will then be discussed. Development strategies such as where to begin and how to proceed, including product acceptance, will also be provided. The section will conclude with an example of third level development efforts and the progress being made for one large, integrated health care system in the USA.

The importance of data collection

Using computerisation to collect information can enhance the evaluation of large amounts of detailed information and provide much more auditing capability than a manual process. As previously mentioned, some organisations have tried to collect manually variance information for analysis during and after the patient's stay, through the medical records department, decision support, cost accounting areas and case managers. A few organisations have had limited success using these methods; for example, the Baptist Health System (Midyette *et al.* 1994) and with John Hopkins (Johnson 1995) and others. But they have soon learned that collecting information in this manner is very expensive, time consuming and sometimes inaccurate. Unless the health care professionals providing the direct patient care are involved in documenting the patient's progress using an on-line structured method, the volume of detailed data needed, with the purest accuracy, cannot be achieved. If automation is the solution, then it must begin at the direct patient care-giver level.

An integrated documentation system has many connotations. It provides the right information for the manager, physicians, other clinicians and administration. But the initial needs must be developed for the direct care-givers first. These are the professionals who will provide the purest detailed information in the most timely and accurate manner. All other disciplines will eventually reap the rewards from the information collected, as the direct care-givers provide it in a real time and proactive manner.

Limitations to current development efforts

Because of the demanding clinical requirements with a system of this nature, and the manual processes being so variable among organisations, it is understandable why integrated clinical solutions are so many years behind other 'business orientated' hospital systems such as financial or billing packages, cost accounting and admission or registration of patients. Only within the past five years have health care organisations in the USA really begun to fund such endeavours. In many institutions the benefits realised by the practice of manual case management have finally given the clinical world the recognition and power to negotiate for IS capital monies and resources that have long been deserved.

In today's environment, many software developers are trying to modify their existing systems to develop an integrated Pathway documentation system that will be a marketable solution. They quickly learn that it simply does not work when installed and are forced back to the drawing board. For example, some developers are using their order management systems (which are often years old) to develop and communicate Pathway information. Most will find this to be a less than satisfactory solution. Clinicians do not, and will not, manage their patients using order processing systems. These systems cannot provide sufficient documentation of what is transpiring with the patient in relation to the expected Pathway outcomes and the patient's progress.

Some developers are attempting to modify their cost accounting systems to provide Pathway management. These systems are primarily revenue and cost based, and thus lack the daily real time documentation characteristics needed to determine when and why variances are occurring. Only detailed concurrent patient documentation, against expected outcomes, will provide the information needed to make effective prospective and retrospective decisions.

Modifications of old solutions are not what is needed to solve today's automation needs. Information system professionals need to abandon their old ideas and start afresh. Pathways of Care are far more complex than simple 'standing orders' when it comes to managing patient care. Old methods of determining efficiency, such as revenue and cost models, will not help in the identification of process problems within complex clinical environments. New ways of looking at documentation and managing patient care are called for, with new applications and databases to support them.

The benefits of an integrated Pathway system

As the clinician provides the necessary documentation, the Pathway system should make use of it appropriately without any additional effort by the clinician. For example, as an abnormal clinical observation or result is recorded, the Pathway system should automatically document a failure in the achievement of expected outcomes, relevant to the observation recorded. This is possible when the applications are designed to guide clinicians to document in a structured manner so that data can be coded automatically as it is collected. This guided documentation should prompt for detailed information only as necessary. It is important not to over-burden the clinician with unnecessary responses that do not pertain to the intervention or outcome in question.

In today's environment there is far too much over-charting, even with automated systems. As interventions are added, revised and removed from the Pathway, they should be automatically communicated to those providing the service as needed. Some interventions may be ancillary orders, consultations, simple messages or nursing tasks. Adjusting the Pathway to add or delete interventions to meet individual patient needs is a routine event and the system must have the intelligence to determine how and when to communicate these changes in interventions. Once again, everyday direct care giver documentation should easily and automatically provide the initiation of such intelligence without additional effort. The system must allow the clinician to document accurately the interventions that are performed. The system should also prompt the clinician to collect detailed information as needed. The clinician should not be forced to determine what information to document, when to document it, and the appropriate policy or process to use, when supplying such documentation. The design of the system must guide the clinician in this effort to ensure accuracy and consistency.

If all interventions necessary to ensuring the outcomes are built into the Pathway and the system prompts the clinician for the appropriate information, then accurate and complete data regarding the patient's course will be recorded. One of the biggest obstacles today to providing workable documentation systems, is the lack of balance in trying to collect the appropriate data detail without overwhelming the clinician in the effort. There is a fine line that must not be breached in this endeavour, or the users of the system will quickly lose respect for it and develop inappropriate shortcuts.

Because all detailed information is located within the Pathway, the system should be able to determine the expected revenue and cost throughout the patient's stay. This information should be available at the intervention and goal level. This is where the various cost accounting systems can be of tremendous benefit. As Pathway interventions are performed for the patient, the system should be able to determine all costs for the day, the phase of care, the procedure, the goal, the intervention and the entire stay. A well designed system will also provide the capability to determine automatically patient acuity. When charting on a fully automated Pathway, using goals with expected outcomes and interventions, the Pathways of Care system should have the ability to determine the significance of the patient's illness without additional care giver evaluation. The evaluation should be performed as charting takes place on the Pathway. Charting against a fully automated Pathway will provide far more accurate acuity levels than are possible with today's systems.

System requirements

Developing an integrated Pathway documentation system will have requirements that are unmatched by other systems currently developed for health care (Fig. 15.2).

A non-negotiable requirement – the direct care giver comes first

The recording of variances from the expected Pathway can be very subjective, resulting in inconsistency of data collection and analysis. Most direct care givers do not understand when variances are occurring, and since it is left up to their interpretation, many may be missed. There are too many documentation requirements, many of which are redundant, and there is too much information to process for maximum productivity and quality in patient care. The system must guide the direct care giver in collecting consistent information as a natural result of their charting processes without adding more effort. The system must be developed to encompass how the care giver provides 'everyday' documentation so that the needed pertinent information will be collected as a natural result.

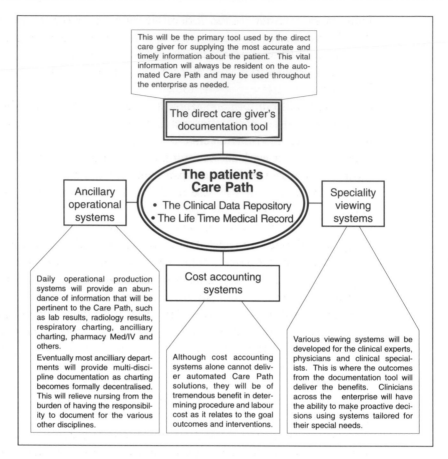

This will be the primary tool used by the direct care giver for supplying the most accurate and timely information about the patient. This vital information will always be resident on the automated Care Path and may be used throughout the enterprise as needed.

The direct care giver's documentation tool

Ancillary operational systems

The patient's Care Path
- The Clinical Data Repository
- The Life Time Medical Record

Speciality viewing systems

Cost accounting systems

Daily operational production systems will provide an abundance of information that will be pertinent to the Care Path, such as lab results, radiology results, respiratory charting, ancilliary charting, pharmacy Med/IV and others.

Eventually most ancilliary departments will provide multi-discipline documentation as charting becomes formally decentralised. This will relieve nursing from the burden of having the responsibility to document for the various other disciplines.

Although cost accounting systems alone cannot deliver automated Care Path solutions, they will be of tremendous benefit in determining procedure and labour cost as it relates to the goal outcomes and interventions.

Various viewing systems will be developed for the clinical experts, physicians and clinical specialists. This is where the outcomes from the documentation tool will deliver the benefits. Clinicians across the enterprise will have the ability to make proactive decisions using systems tailored for their special needs.

Fig. 15.2   The conceptual view of the automated documentation system.

General system requirements

The following system requirements should be included in the development of any integrated Pathway documentation system (Favor & Ricks 1995):

- The system must maintain strict relationships between Pathway components such as categories, phases, goal outcomes, interventions, and problems.
- The Pathway will serve as the focal point for all patient documentation, whether it is clinical or financial. The Pathway of Care is the complete plan of care, therefore it must be at the heart of the medical record. Ultimately it will form the structure around which the lifetime medical record should be built.
- The system must have the ability to store all relevant clinical information indefinitely. The system must have the means to retrieve historical

Pathway information just as it does for current, or active, patient stay data. Those analysing this information should only need to access one view for all information. No one should ever have to view Pathway data in an active format, an historical format and an archived format that each look and feel different. With today's technologies it is reasonable to expect, and demand, all information (no matter its age) to be resident on the database with the same format (although retrieval of archived data may be a little slower than active data files).

- The system must work across multiple care entities in a truly enterprise setting. Although the data may span many entities it should be resident in one, and only one, database platform that best fits the health care system's needs. Many developers claim to support a multiple entity enterprise system, but in fact they are simply copying their software many times (based on the number of corporate entities) and storing each as a separate file structure on the same computer in different regions. This is done because it is time consuming and expensive to enhance existing legacy systems to truly function in a multiple facility enterprise structure. This method of providing multiple facility computing does not make Pathways easily accessible across a corporate enterprise.

- The system must use a widely accepted, standard, relational database. This should be a database structure that allows access by multiple entities without changing databases. The database should have the flexibility to support the use of popular decision support tools without using additional data extraction processes.

- All charted information should be coded in such a manner that operational reports and decision support personnel can accurately generate information as necessary using any common report-writing tool. Coding of charted information will be the key to successful data collection and retrieval. The days of 'free text' Pathway information have passed. Every component of the Pathway should have a unique coding scheme. All charting detail must be automatically coded as it is entered to allow optimum flexibility in the passing of data for reporting.

- The system should have the highest usage of all health care information systems. The amount of information and transactions will exceed that of most systems currently used in clinical practice. It is of the utmost importance that response time be sub-second, meaning that the movement from screen to screen should be less than a second. In other words, the system must be extremely fast in response to user commands to enter and display data. No time-pressured clinician wants to wait even a second for the system to respond as information is entered or reviewed. Sub-second response time should be a non-negotiable agreement before implementation begins. The system will have more users bidding for its resources than that of any clinical system used today, but response time cannot be compromised or it will not be acceptable to clinicians.

Development strategies

Where to begin

Developing a system that provides the direct care giver with the benefit of fast, easy, automated documentation should be the first priority of the development and implementation project cycle. Maintaining this objective, whether it is an in-house developer or marketing vendor, gives the best chances for success.

The development effort may include the integration of the following documentation features:

- Admission physical assessments
- Shift assessments
- Charting observations against interventions, treatments and procedures
- Vital signs, intake and output
- Admission history
- Discharge history and planning
- Medication, intravenous administration charting
- Managing treatments and procedures (adding, deleting and modifying)
- Documenting the patient's progress against the expected outcomes
- Documenting patient specific notes

Providing such a documentation tool is extremely complicated and forces integration with a variety of functions that must be easy and straightforward in use. The following may be only some of the functions which should be included:

- The ability to build predefined Pathways and the ability to graphically print them
- The ability to assign Pathways of Care to patients
- The ability to adjust all goal outcomes and interventions to individualise the patient's care
- The ability to document goal outcomes
- The ability to document clinical observations and results against the interventions
- The ability to progress the patient through each phase of care
- The ability to extend, or repeat, a phase of care when necessary
- The ability to notify ancillary departments of interventions appropriate to their area, and manage associated charges and costs

- The ability to overlay a primary Pathway with secondary Pathways and care protocols for drugs or special treatments
- Operational reports for direct care givers, case managers and administration
- All reports accompanied by similar on-line displays
- Appropriate documentation to perform decision support reporting for trending and analysis

Future phases

Installation of the first phases of system development will give the direct care giver a complete documentation tool for their everyday needs. If designed correctly, the documentation tool will be the primary collector of all detailed data needed from the care giver's point of view. All other phases of the system development will function as spin-offs of this base documentation tool and will be seen as enhancements to the applications by the primary care giver. It is important to remember to continue to enhance the first phases, using the direct care giver's input, as future phases are rolled out. The following are future phases that should be relatively easy to implement once the primary documentation system is installed and the users become acclimatised to it.

Continue to improve the documentation process, seeking new ways to provide for easier, faster charting. As the system is initially installed, discrepancies between the theory of practice and the design will become apparent in the reality of everyday clinical use. Developers may perform a variety of tests and evaluations for months before final implementation, but improvements will always be necessary following installation as the clinicians begin to use the system in a live environment. Developers should plan to spend at least six to twelve months on enhancements, adjustments, even redesigning portions of the system, but at the same time they should not hold up the continued development of future phases. Executive management needs to understand this commitment throughout the project. Automation of Pathways into a fully integrated documentation system is going boldly on a risky new adventure, which requires prototyping and constant change to accomplish a long term successful implementation.

Bring the outcomes and the interventions closer together. Interventions are being charted for the purpose of achieving the outcomes that are predefined for the patient. Therefore the system should have the intelligence to know when the outcomes are achieved or not, based on the results and observations recorded against the interventions. For example, if a clinician is using the system to chart the patient's vital signs from an intervention on the Pathway, and the heart rate is recorded as 82, then the system should perform the following:

(1)   Determine the Pathway the patient is on
(2)   Determine the phase of care within the Pathway
(3)   Find the goal outcome within the phase of care that relates to heart rate and automatically chart whether the outcome was achieved or not
(4)   Print or display the result on the appropriate reports or work lists

Today's clinicians are constantly 'over-recording' and 'double-charting'. A well designed system should reduce this through the automatic communication of ancillary orders, as interventions are added to the Pathway or the patient progresses; through receiving results and clinical observations from ancillary systems such as laboratory, radiology, respiratory, physical therapy and pharmacy and directing them to outcomes and interventions on the Pathway; and through automatically determining patient acuity based on the Pathway record, and providing easy migration for archiving data so that the existing system functionality continues to be used to review and chart related information as the patient returns for follow up visits.

User acceptance of the Pathway of Care documentation system

Not enough can be said concerning the requirements for acceptance of such a Pathway system within the clinical community. This system will dramatically change everything related to the clinician's documentation process and how it is viewed in the record by all clinicians and physicians. Neither an IS department nor a software vendor alone can truly support the installation of an automated Pathway system without the 'buy-in' of the clinicians of all disciplines using it. Change of this magnitude will generate much controversy that must be dealt with at all levels of management.

For the first six to twelve months of the initial installation of the system, technical and clinical support should be available at all times. This support should be routinely visible at the clinical site by the actual users of the system on all shifts. This means on the unit, in the charting room, at the work station, in the lunch room, at the bedside. Only when the end user knows that there is that level of commitment, will they help to overcome the obstacles to making the project successful and identifying the enhancements needed.

An example of third level automation

At Baptist Health System (BHS) in Birmingham, Alabama, a project is underway to develop an integrated case management documentation system (Favor & Ricks 1995). BHS is a non-profit corporate entity made up of 11 hospitals with over 2000 licensed acute care beds, multiple clinics, home health agencies, and retirement homes as well as other related corporate entities. Case management was identified as a major corporate strategic initiative for improving patient care and holding down costs in 1993. Automation was seen as critical to maximise the benefits of the case management process.

In November 1993 a detailed analysis of the current manual system and the automation requirements was performed and a proposal developed. This proposal was initially presented to the consulting firm of KPMG Peat Marwick and then to the management executive committee (MEC) of BHS. The MEC approved the 1.5 million dollar project, which provided for in-house development of an integrated case management documentation system. The system was to be developed and implemented in six overlapping phases, each of which were estimated to require six months.

The project uses a prototype approach with close input and direction provided by the staff and case managers using the system. The authors are the development team's technical and clinical co-leaders. Initially the team included three programmers, but two more have recently been added to aid developments and they have integrated medication and intravenous administration charting.

At the time of writing, the project is in the fourth phase. The project has consistently been able to remain ahead of schedule through each phase. In the first phase, case managers were able to build their Care Maps® on the computer and display, print and modify them. In the second phase they were able to assign a map, progress the patient across the phases of care and enter variances. They were also able to print a census of their patients showing the most recent variances. In the third phase, the open heart progressive care nursing staff were able to manage their patients using the Care Maps® and document both outcomes and interventions. The nursing staff had a high initial acceptance of the product and it was installed in the open heart intensive care unit.

As the fourth phase of the project was developed, which provided for the integration of the recording of assessments and more detailed charting of treatments and procedures, there has been increasing dissension concerning the project direction. As with all projects involving such a magnitude of change, management is having to reconsider many issues related to on-line medical records and the ability of middle management to incorporate and adjust to a new approach. This reaction should be expected by any vendor or organisation attempting to provide leading edge automation.

Level 4 – the future

As standardisation and automation of clinical documentation become more refined and are integrated with Pathways of Care, the vision of the future will take shape with two major benefits. The first is the ability to provide automatic notification of patient problems ('alerts') by the computer. The second is the development of a variety of specialised clinical workstations to assist physicians, ancillary clinical specialists and case managers to see what is currently transpiring with their individual patients, as well as providing the capability for viewing and graphing trends for groups of patients. These are the ultimate goals for developing an integrated Pathway system and only when these benefits are realised will true improvements in patient care and real control of costs be possible.

Automatic notification of potential variances (also known as on-line 'alerts' or decision support), can only be achieved by the use of a highly structured, centralised, relational database. As clinicians record care, the system must be designed to collect the data in a very structured manner. This allows combinations of data to be analysed and an 'alert' to be generated. At a very simple level such an 'alert' might consist of failing the expected outcome of a heart rate between 60–100 beats/minute. A more complicated 'alert' might combine a drug the patient is on with the clinical observation of an elevated heart rate to notify the clinician immediately of a potential problem related to the drug. Information on clinical observations, laboratory work and drugs, when collected in a centralised database, can be analysed real time, and 'alerts' issued only if the data is standardised.

Another part of achieving on-line clinical alerting is providing a system in which most 'alerts' can easily be built by the clinical experts themselves. The vast majority of the 'alerts' are relatively straightforward and only a minor number are so complex as to require extensive programming. To easily build 'alerts', there must be an integrated, centralised, relational database attached to a clinical workstation which provides the clinician with the menu driven capability to combine the data elements needed. The clinician would be able to select the data elements, the relational symbols needed (such as $>$, $<$ or $=$) and enter the appropriate ranges, to which the system provides the codes to build the 'alert'. Although this may sound like technology that is years away, in reality it is achievable today provided the base systems are properly built. Leading health care organisations will achieve this ability within the next couple of years.

A final benefit to automation is the specialised clinical workstation. This consists of clinical applications specifically designed to provide on-line, current graphical data to specialised users. Where today's leading organisations provide decision support with reports that take weeks and months for clinicians to receive, and consume expensive resources to provide, tomorrow's specialised workstations will put clinicians in the driving seat.

This too will be possible sooner than most would think, but once again it requires automated documentation systems which are integrated and highly structured with centrally stored data.

A system that notifies the clinician as things are going wrong and instantaneously provides graphics of current patient outcomes, as well as trends for combinations of patients in an easy to use real time display, is the goal of today's automation efforts. To achieve such benefits will challenge both health care organisations and information systems specialists. These benefits will happen, but their accomplishment will take massive re-engineering of today's manual documentation systems. It will not be vendors that lead the way in this endeavour, although they will benefit. It will be health care organisations with visionary management, as well as clinicians and information systems professionals working together to provide the design, development, installation, and on-going support of such systems. These organisations will supply the people, the capital and the risk-taking environment that will allow them to make the mistakes and learn the lessons necessary to push forward to the next level of automation in health care.

Summary

The challenge facing automation efforts for Pathways of Care today is to bring data together in a manner that helps clinicians to focus on the patient's progress or lack of it: where are the problems occurring? This is where integrating documentation within Pathways can truly be of benefit to the clinician's efforts in providing quality patient care. As Zander (1993) put it: 'products that allow concurrent management and documentation of care to drive all other information will win the race for market share'. This includes integrated documentation of results, observations, treatments, outcomes, orders, acuity, cost, and even the use of supplies. It must provide for staff to follow patients across the continuum of care, from acute care, to skilled nursing care, to home or community care, rehabilitation, outpatient, and physician follow-up. This is a daunting task for information systems professionals, requiring careful development from both a system operations perspective and long range IS strategic planning. It is possible to accomplish, but it will take tremendous effort, executive vision, and very well thought out long range planning. The race is on. Victory will go to those organisations with the combined executive, clinical, and information systems vision and resolve to institute a long range, evolutionary process to change the way care is documented in support of an integrated case management process across the continuum of care.

References

Favor, G. & Ricks, R. (1995) Mapping care one step at a time. *Healthcare Informatics*, May, 32–8.

HIMSS/HP Survey Results (1995) Special Report. *Healthcare Informatics*. May.

Johnson, K. (1995) Pediatrician leads case management. *Issues & Outcomes*, May/June.

Midyette, P., Meisler, N., & Ricks, R. (1994) Computerised Variance Analysis Management. Poster presentation at a meeting of the American Association of Critical Care Nurses, Atlanta, Georgia.

Zander, K. (1993) Dear I/S vendor. *Computers in Healthcarre*, June, 34.

Introduction

The National Health Service (NHS) is probably the single most powerful idea to have been conceived in Britain this century. Its aim was, and still is, to provide health care for all according to need, and for that care to be free at the point of delivery. The expectation was to provide everything to everyone, eventually resulting in a healthier population that would then require fewer resources in the long term. However, this vision did not anticipate the dramatic changes in medical technology, the increasing public interest in health care, subsequent demographic patterns and changes in service provision.

Fifty or so years down the road the continued development of the NHS has produced many dilemmas. These have been brought to a head in the latest set of reforms, with various debates starting to take place in the public arena. Hard questions are being asked about equity and access to health care; about clinical care needing to be based on scientific evidence; about outcomes of care that can be truly measurable and about high value for the quality of services provided.

The white paper *Working For Patients* (DoH 1989), made these changes explicit, enabling the separation of functions between the purchasing and the provision of health care. This has allowed health authorities to concentrate on assessing the health needs of the populations they serve, and to decide how best they should be met. As this function has developed and matured, certain issues which hitherto had lain undiscovered have been brought into the open.

It has never been possible to provide limitless resources for health care, although the NHS has sometimes behaved as if it were. As we approach the end of the twentieth century, resources have become tighter and public expectations more demanding, accelerated by the Patient's Charter (1991). Purchasers of health care have had to ensure that the services they commission come nearer to reflecting the needs of their populations. In parallel, there has been a shift of focus from the primary aim of curing the sick to the achievement of health gain.

The need for comparative measures of performance and quality therefore become increasingly pressing, and all the more so when concepts of care in new and different settings have had to be explored, initiated and backed up by sound clinical evidence.

National priorities in the UK, such as the Health of the Nation (DoH 1992) and the Research and Development Strategy (EL(94)74) have attempted to provide a focused framework for the NHS. However, these policies and initiatives require reliable translation to the local scene. With such diverse and increasing requirements (especially as the role of the regional health authorities diminishes and finally disappears) purchasers need an effective mechanism for achieving this.

The responsibilities of purchasers

In order to understand the tasks required of purchasers of health care, it is necessary to clarify their roles and responsibilities (EL(94)79). These are:

- To implement national health policy
- To assess health needs of their local populations
- To place value for money contracts for health care
- To integrate primary and secondary strategies
- To develop primary care

This has facilitated the merging of functions of district health authorities and family health service authorities into one statutory authority for commissioning across the primary/secondary setting (Health Authorities Act 1995). This is a vast agenda requiring a systematic and co-ordinated approach to the planning of health care. Pathways of Care could be a key mechanism for achieving this major task.

Assessment of health needs

Assessment of health needs of a defined population (a function traditionally carried out by Public Health) involves review of current service provision (staff, equipment, clinics, etc.), taking into account the education and training needs of the health service personnel, and matching provision with the requirements of the population.

A number of factors, as well as central initiatives need to be incorporated into this process. The effect on medical manpower of various reports, for example the reduction in junior doctors' hours (NHSME 1991) and the Calman Report (DoH 1993) on specialist medical training, will greatly influence service provision. Fears have been expressed concerning fragmentation and poor communication as the numbers of staff decrease and the changeover of staff is increased as a result of the implementation of these recommendations. There is also a need to ensure that the expensive resource of a consultant is used to best effect at the right time and place.

By providing a defined, consistent and agreed method of working, Pathways can improve communication and quantify more precisely the type of clinical care to be provided. Compliance with new systems is more likely to be adhered to if they have been generated by the very team who are required to implement the changed method of working, rather than having the system imposed upon them from management. Thus it is the clinicians themselves who must be central to the development and implementation of a system such as Pathways of Care.

Other clinical professions are not exempt. Within the nursing development agenda, Pathways could identify and aid decisions with regard to education and training (UKCC 1990), good practice, clinical outcomes and audit (NHSME 1993). For example, in skill mix exercises, Pathways could clarify the delineation of tasks requiring a qualified clinical professional and those which could be provided by a generic worker. The latter, once identified, could then be trained through the National Vocational Qualification (NVQ) training scheme. The health professionals would thus be free to develop and refine their own clinical skills and expertise.

Nurses are facing a challenge with the development of the nurse practitioner role (STRHA 1994). This specialised nursing role is defined by the ability to diagnose conditions, initiate treatment and make referrals to relevant specialists. This role has, in my opinion, its best potential for growth in primary care, by working alongside the general practitioner (GP), with a proportion of the GP's workload being transferred to the nurse practitioner.

It is essential that agreed guidelines are drawn up for the functioning of this role, and with professionals in primary care tending to work in teams already, the Pathway provides a useful framework for this.

Placing contracts for health care

As the contracting system has developed, there has been a recognition of the increasing difficulty in measuring the performance or outcomes of care for the same speciality or service across different providers, making it hard to make comparisons. For example, prices for inpatient work for a particular speciality cannot always be compared because, due to the variations in care provision between the different providers, the purchasers are not comparing like with like. The use of healthcare resource groups (HRGs) has begun to tackle this problem, with orthopaedic, ophthalmology and gynaecology conditions and procedures being costed within related resource groupings in the first instance. Later general surgery, ear nose and throat surgery and urology were added to the list of HRGs (EL(95)79).

It is noticeable that the medical specialities are absent from the HRGs selected thus far. Medical conditions are the hardest to quantify using this method of costing, as the course of treatment is far less predictable than in surgery, and depends on a number of factors relating to the concurrent conditions that the medical patient may have. Pathways enable the collection of data in this area as a number of Pathways have been drawn up across the country for the more common medical conditions (myocardial infarction, stroke, asthma, deep vein thrombosis, etc.). Thus Pathways of Care have a role to play in assisting the costing process for health care contracts, as they set out the anticipated course of treatment for specific conditions (see Chapter 14).

Clinical audit

Purchasers are scrutinising clinical care, and demanding audits of the care provided and the clinical outcomes of treatments. No longer can audit be performed at the whim of the consultant as was often done with traditional medical audit. Increasingly clinical audit is serving as a mechanism for purchasers to check and ensure that the clinical processes of all disciplines involved in care are appropriate and effective, and if they are not, to ensure that changes in clinical practice do occur to improve the situations. Purchasers require as much robust clinical evidence as possible on the health services they commission, so that they may be confident that they have secured the best care for their population.

How effective are provider unit's clinical audit programmes at improving clinical practices and patient care? As health authorities become more sophisticated in their examination of clinical audit, the use of variance data from the Pathways becomes increasingly important to provide objective information on the care delivered. Evidence-based commissioning is the provision of services that are the best possible clinical practice according to research evidence, and the prevention of procedures of dubious clinical value. Audit data and information from the analysis of variances from Pathways will assist the purchasing authorities in their decisions on where best care is provided.

Research and development

Clinical research sometimes reveals that long established methods of treatment are of doubtful value, yet the practices still continue. The implementation of research into actual service delivery seems to be a slow process. Some successes have occurred; for example, the Getting Research into Practice (GRIP) initiative launched by Oxford Regional Health Authority in 1993. The projects covered were:

- Use of corticosteroids in pre-term delivery
- Use of therapeutic dilatation and curettage in women under the age of 40
- Use of surgery for children with suspected glue ear
- Management of services for stroke patients

Research has now been commissioned through the national research and development programme to investigate different methods of integrating research evidence into clinical practice. Nevertheless, currently very little of the vast amount of research performed is used as a vehicle for change in service delivery with the resulting improvement in health outcomes. This may be because of inadequate awareness amongst the decision makers; it could be a case of 'old habits die hard', and a lack of familiarity with new practices. Pathways of Care have the capacity to provide a safe environment to test out the research in active clinical situations which are under the control of those who are providing the care. There may even be instances where Pathways can provide a pointer for where further research into clinical practice is required.

Risk management

In April 1995 the Central Fund for Clinical Negligence was set up (EL(95)40). The responsibility for clinical negligence was transferred to NHS trusts and provider units on 1 April 1991, although health authorities have had to bear the costs of claims occurring prior to that time. At the time of writing, claims from before April 1991 are still filtering through to purchasers with a trend of increasing cost of settlements.

This should soon cease to have a direct impact on health authorities, although the indirect effects of providers' units taking on the responsibility will continue to be felt. These appear in the guise of higher prices transferred to purchasers as providers seek to cover their costs. There has been a rise in consumer awareness, expectations of clinical services, and complaints about poor patient care over recent years. Clearly by not getting it right first time, with the resultant claims made on care providers, the question of value for money will be raised in addition to the quality of patient care.

Providers will come under pressure from purchasers to demonstrate good clinical risk management, and Pathways will facilitate this requirement by demonstrating the presence of agreed clinical guidelines for care and an effective monitoring system rolled into one model of care delivery.

Integration of primary and secondary care

The philosophy behind the new combined health authorities (Health Authorities Act 1995), is to ensure the integration of primary and secondary care. This is most needed in the management of chronic diseases, such as diabetes, asthma, epilepsy, stroke, etc., which encompass fragmented areas such as prescribing and discharge procedures, as well as communication between agencies like social services.

The task of drawing up and agreeing packages of care is hugely complex and probably best initiated through the application of Pathways of Care. Using this technique purchasers, providers and GPs can work together to formulate their services together, in a non-confrontational and non-threatening manner. Small Pathways may be produced in different settings, concentrating on particular episodes of the overall continuum of care. These can then be brought together to form a larger Pathway which could then form the basis of the total package of care. This could then form the contract currency – the element describing the health care to be provided.

For example, drawing up a service for diabetic patients could include a number of Pathways for the different clinical settings involved (Fig. 16.1). Diabetics in the community setting would be grouped according to their needs (newly diagnosed insulin dependent diabetic, or non-insulin diabetic with complications etc.), then they would have contact with various professionals at a variety of clinics in the community, from the practice nurse to

---

Management of diabetics in the community:
- Newly diagnosed diabetics (insulin and non-insulin dependent)
- Diagnosed diabetics
- Diabetics with complications.

Management of diabetics in hospital:
- Emergency admission
- Planned admission for stabilisation
- Treatment of advanced complications
- Joint clinics (e.g. with maternity, ophthalmology, nephrology, etc.)
- Paediatric diabetics.

Fig. 16.1 Diabetes Pathways.

the chiropodist. Diabetics in hospital would again be grouped accordingly, with Pathways for children, pregnant diabetics, emergency admission with diabetic ketoacidosis, and so on. These individual Pathways would then develop together to form a service for diabetics in that district that crosses the primary/secondary interface. Local situations would demand local approaches to such services, and this would need to be reflected in the local Pathways constructed.

A similar process could be used for prescribing and discharge issues between hospitals, community services, primary health care teams and social services.

A primary care led NHS

The 1991 NHS reforms (DoH 1989) brought into play a new type of purchaser, the GP fundholder (GPFH). The GPFH uses their skills as a clinician to purchase health care direct from providers of their own choice, rather than relying on the local purchasing authority to do this for them. As the range of services to be purchased by GPFHs has expanded, so has their responsibility. This has been formalised in the GP Fundholder Accountability Framework (EL(94)79).

At the launch of this document there was also reference to health authorities enabling all GPs to become more closely involved in commissioning, to be part of a 'primary care led NHS'. This has set the scene for the development of locality purchasing or locality commissioning, that is, GPs coming together in small groups to commission a defined set of services for their local population, facilitated by the purchasing authority.

The GP Fundholder Accountability Framework sets out the four main areas of responsibility required of GPFHs:

Management accountability

- Preparation of an annual practice plan
- Signalling major shifts in purchasing intentions
- Preparation of an annual performance report
- Review of performance with the health authority within the national framework.

Accountability to patients and the wider public

- Publishing information (annual practice plan, performance report, etc.)
- Involving patients in service planning
- Ensuring an effective complaints system.

Financial accountability

- Preparation of annual accounts for independent audit
- Providing monthly information for monitoring by the health authority
- Securing health authority agreements to use of savings
- Stating planned contribution to the local efficiency targets set by the NHS Executive.

Clinical and professional accountability

- Participating in the clinical audit of general medical services activities
- Ensuring appropriate clinical audit of purchased hospital and community health care.

Clearly, responsibilities could seem overwhelming to fundholders who are grappling with increasing demands on their time as clinicians as well as purchasers. Pathways could provide a helpful tool in a number areas; for example, with administrative processes such as the production of the business plan and the purchasing intentions, and all the co-ordination that these require. Internal administrative systems could also benefit from the application of the Pathway tool; for example, dealing with complaints procedures.

Pathways of Care could also be well utilised in the further development of clinical audit in primary care and in the combined interface audit between hospitals, community and GP services.

Working with other agencies

The NHS clearly does not work in isolation. As the drive to maintain people in the community for as long as possible continues, close collaboration with other agencies such as social services and the voluntary or private sector becomes vital. Although the NHS through the Community Care Act (DoH 1990) places the responsibility for community care with local authority social services departments, this still requires full partnership with local health authorities. Communication is of utmost importance when the achievement of common goals is the central aim, and when there are shared working practices. Pathways of Care could facilitate this by strengthening the link between health and social care, as well as involving other voluntary organisations, patients and carers.

The Care Programme Approach (HC(90)23, HC(90)24) is another requirement for joint co-operation between a number of agencies when planning packages of care for people with mental health problems. In its short history, the ideal set out in this document has broken down, and in a number of cases communication has been cited as a causal factor of the failure (SETRHA 1994). If used effectively, Pathways of Care could go some way to remedy the lack of effective communication between agencies and across care provider units, and thus ensure that the risk of untoward incidents is minimised.

Into the future with Pathways of Care

This chapter has made reference to a number of policies and central initiatives which, although they have laudable aims, do not seem to work out so well in practice for many reasons. The potential link between the philosophy and usefulness of Pathways and these policies have been identified in both clinical and non-clinical settings. The 'bottom-up' approach in the establishment of Pathways by those professionals actively involved in the delivery of health and social care, is the strength of this methodology.

The process has added value in that clinical standards and guidelines can be incorporated according to local circumstances, thereby optimising patient care. The Pathways can be developed into packages of care, a contract currency which includes appropriate standards of care, clinical audit and future research and development of services for client groups or specific conditions. These packages of care will then have an inherent updating mechanism as further good practice comes to light. Furthermore, Pathways of Care provide a controlled process of examining the clinical and cost effectiveness of health services, which will ultimately be beneficial for the patient.

The consistency of approach and the precise definition of the type of care provided through the use of Pathways, with the monitoring of clinical outcomes and use of resources by different providers, allow purchasers to make more accurate comparisons of similar services. Providers who are able to demonstrate clinical and cost effective care for the best health gain, make the process of placing contracts relatively more simple.

The need to demonstrate evidence-based commissioning grows stronger. This will surely accelerate as the purchasers of health care become more sophisticated, with the involvement of GPs (both fundholders and non-fundholders). With such clinical input, questions regarding the effectiveness and appropriateness of clinical care will inevitably be raised. By providing a true clinical approach to care that can be understood by purchasers and GPs, Pathways are probably the most powerful tool for leading the clinical development of health services.

With the development of health services being dependent on a political process, the configuration of the types of purchasers in the market will continue to change. Fundholding may be transformed into locality commissioning, and the role of district purchasing authorities for placing contracts will probably diminish. However, there will remain a need to plan strategically for health care, and to target priority groups as resources continue to be outstripped by demand. The push to ensure the most clinically effective health care will become stronger as the practices of healthcare delivery advance, particularly as technology proves to be increasingly expensive, and consumer satisfaction more demanding. In this environment, Pathways of Care are ripe for development.

References

DoH (1993) *Hospital Doctors: Training for the Future*, Working Group on Specialist Medical Training, chaired by K. Calman. HMSO, London.

DoH (1989) *Working For Patients*. HMSO, London.

DoH (1991) *The Patient's Charter*. HMSO, London.

DoH (1992) *The Health of the Nation: A Strategy for Health in England*. HMSO, London.

DoH (1990) *The NHS and the Community Care Act*. HMSO, London.

EL(94)74. *Improving the Effectiveness of the NHS*. September 1994.

EL(94)79. *Developing NHS Purchasing and GP Fundholding*. October 1994.

EL(95)79. *The Use of Costed HRGs in the 1996/7 Contracting Cycle*. July 1995.

EL(95)40 *The Central Fund for Clinical Negligence*. 1995.

HC(90)23 & HC(90)24. *The Care Programme Approach. 1990.*

SETRHA (South East Thames Regional Health Authority) *Report of the Inquiry into the Care and Treatment of Christopher Clunis*. Chaired by J. Ritchie QC. HMSO, London.

STRHA (South Thames Regional Health Authority) (1994) *Evaluation of Nurse Practitioner Pilot Projects*. Touche Ross Management Consultants, London.

NHSME (1993) *A Vision for the Future*. HMSO, London.

NHSME (1991) *Junior Doctors; the New Deal*. HMSO, London.

UKCC (1990) *Post-registration Education and Practice Project*. United Kingdom Central Council for Nursing, Midwifery and Health Visiting, London.

Index